ERRATA

page 111: In sub-heading of Table II read for μCi : nCi.
Idem in note to Table II (2x).

page 113: In caption for figure 3 read for μCi : nCi.

page 194: In line 11 from bottom read for μCi : nCi.

Biological Effects of ^{224}Ra

This symposium was organized by the

Commission of the European Communities,
Directorate-General Research, Science and Education,
Biology, Radiation Protection and Medical Research,
Brussels, Belgium

and the

Gesellschaft für Strahlen- und Umweltforschung mbH,
Neuherberg/München, Federal Republic of Germany

Programme Committee:

W. Gössner, Neuherberg/München
O. Hug, Neuherberg/München
C.W. Mays, Salt Lake City, Utah
R. Mole, Harwell
F. Schales †, Frankfurt

Scientific Secretary:

W.A. Müller, Neuherberg/München

Local Committee:

E. Parchwitz, Neuherberg/München

Neuherberg/München, September 20-21, 1976
Publication date: January 1978

Biological Effects of ^{224}Ra

Benefit and Risk of Therapeutic Application

Proceedings of the Second Symposium at
Neuherberg/München, September 20-21, 1976

Editors

W. A. Müller

Institut für Biologie,
Gesellschaft für Strahlen- und Umweltforschung m.b.H.,
Neuherberg/München, Federal Republic of Germany

and

H. G. Ebert

Commission of the European Communities,
Directorate-General Research, Science and Education
Biology, Radiation Protection and Medical Research.

Martinus Nijhoff Medical Division - The Hague/Boston 1978
for
The Commission of the European Communities

Publication arranged by
Commission of the European Communities,
Directorate-General Scientific and Technical Information
and Information Management, Luxembourg

EUR 5867e

Softcover reprint of the hardcover 1st edition 1978

Publication date: January 1978

ISBN-13:978-94-009-9730-1 e-ISBN-13:978-94-009-9728-8
DOI: 10.1007/978-94-009-9728-8

Abstract

The Second Symposium on the Biological Effects of ^{224}Ra, held at Neuherberg, was focused on two topical aspects of radiation protection. One aspect was the long-term effects of high-LET ionizing radiations on man and the quantitative data involved in risk assessment at low doses. The evaluation of epidemiological studies and experimental research was discussed in order to provide facts and figures contributing to an objective assessment of the radiation hazard from incorporated radionuclides.

The other aspect was that of radiation protection in medicine. In the case of ^{224}Ra treatment of ankylosing spondylitis the questions of benefit and risk of this therapeutic use of ionizing radiations were discussed, the aim being to achieve the therapeutic effect while reducing radiation exposure - and therefore the hazard - to a minimum. The proceedings contain the complete texts of 23 papers as well as the final round table discussions.

Table of contents

		page
H.G. Ebert W.A. Müller	Preface	1
C.W. Mays	On the scientific work of Fritz Schales	5
W. Gössner	Opening adress	7
Session I	Chairman: W. Gössner	
F.W. Hartl	Zur Klinik der ankylosierenden Spondylitis (Morbus Bechterew)	11
F. Schilling	Pathology and radiology of ankylosing spondylitis	19
Session II	Chairmen: A. Bertrand, B. Windeyer	
W. Koch	Indication for ^{224}Ra-therapy in ankylosing spondylitis	21
F. Schales	Problems and results of a new follow-up study - ^{224}Ra in adult ankylosing spondylitis patients	30
C.W. Mays	Addendum to the previous paper: Risk to bone from present ^{224}Ra therapy	37
O. Delikan	Quality control in the production process and purity of ^{224}Ra for injection	44
E. Schmitt	Therapeutical results in a follow-up study ^{224}Ra-therapy of ankylosing spondylitis	50
B. Windeyer	X-ray therapy in the treatment of ankylosing spondylitis	60
Session III	Chairmen: J. Martin, C. Winkler	
I. Bahous	Radiosynoviorthesis: Local treatment of rheumatoid arthritis	71
A. Bertrand J. Martin C. Hocquard	Comparison of the efficacy of ^{224}Ra and other radio-isotopes in the treatment of rheumatoid arthritis	79

B. Wallner W.A. Müller	Experimental data on the injection of ^{224}Ra into the knee-joint of rats and rabbits	87
W. Koch	Intravenous injection of ^{224}Ra in Morbus Paget	95
Session IV	Chairman: H. Spiess	
H. Spiess	Clinical experiences concerning late effects and risks of ^{224}Ra	102
V. Dvořák et al.	Osteogenic sarcomas in mice after ^{224}Ra or ^{226}Ra administrations	109
V. Kofránek et al.	Biological effects of ^{224}Ra and ^{226}Ra and their relative radiotoxicity in mice	120
A. Luz W.A. Müller W. Gössner O. Hug	The dependence of late effects in mice on the temporal distribution of skeletal α-doses from ^{224}Ra and ^{227}Th	135
K.H. Marquart W. Gössner	Histopathology of early effects of ^{224}Ra on bone tissue	149
V. Erfle K.H. Marquart	Expression of type C RNA virus particles in ^{224}Ra-induced osteosarcomas	158
Session V	Chairman: G.W. Dolphin	
C.W. Mays H. Spiess	Bone sarcoma risks to man from ^{224}Ra, ^{226}Ra and ^{239}Pu	168
G.W. Dolphin	Problems in radiological protection involving α-emitters in bone	182
P.G. Groer J.H. Marshall	A model for the induction of bone cancer by ^{224}Ra	201
J. Martin A. Bertrand	Methodological aspect of epidemiological inquiries in clinical radiobiology	210
H. Roux et al.	Notre experience du ^{224}Ra dans le traitement de la spondylarthrite ankylosante	212

Round Table Discussion I Moderator: C.W. Mays
Risk evaluation of ankylosing spondylitis therapy 215

Round Table Discussion II Moderator: W. Koch
Clinical results of ankylosing spondylitis therapy 223

R.H. Mole Concluding remarks 230

List of participants 233

Preface

Under an association contract linking the Commission of the European Communities and the Gesellschaft für Strahlen- und Umweltforschung mbH, a research programme on the pathogenesis of somatic radiation damage has been under way for a number of years. Experimental research on long-term radiation effects following the incorporation of bone-seeking radionuclides and an epidemiological study of the consequences for patients treated with ^{224}Ra for therapeutical reasons have been among the main features of the work. The research carried out on tumor induction in the low dose range and for low dose rates is particularly important as regards assessing the radiation hazard to man.

The second Symposium on the biological effects of ^{224}Ra, held at Neuherberg, provided a welcome opportunity to take stock of what has been achieved so far and to discuss the own research efforts in an international setting. The discussions focussed on two topical aspects of radiation protection.

One aspect was the long-term effects of high-LET ionizing radiations on man and the quantitative data involved in risk assessment at low doses. The epidemiological studies and experimental research carried out under the association contract should provide facts and figures for an objective assessment of the radiation hazards from incorporated radionuclides, which is one of the fundamental and controversial problems of the nuclear energy debate.

The other aspect was that of radiation protection in medicine. In the case of ^{224}Ra treatment of ankylosing spondylitis the question about benefit and risk of this therapeutic use of ionizing radiations was discussed. In the light of the results presented, it should be possible, when the appropriate indications are met, to achieve the therapeutic effect while reducing radiation exposure - and therefore the hazard - to a minimum.

These two topics are closely related and it was a 'bonus' of the Symposium that both clinical experiences and radiobiological research results were presented and discussed with a view to clarifying the questions involved.

H.G. EBERT W.A. MüLLER

Vorwort

Die Kommission der Europäischen Gemeinschaften und die Gesellschaft für Strahlen- und Umweltforschung mbH führen seit mehreren Jahren im Rahmen eines Assoziationsvertrages ein Forschungsprogramm über die Pathogenese der somatischen Strahlenschäden durch. Experimentelle Untersuchungen über die Spätschäden nach Inkorporation osteotroper Radionuklide und epidemiologische Studien über die Folgen einer ^{224}Ra-Behandlung von Patienten gehören mit zu den Schwerpunkten der Arbeiten der Assoziation. Von besonderer Bedeutung im Hinblick auf die Strahlengefährdung des Menschen ist dabei das Studium der Tumorinduktion im Bereich niedriger Dosen und Dosisleistungen.

Es war somit eine willkommene Gelegenheit, das 2. Symposium über die biologischen Effekte von ^{224}Ra in Neuherberg zu organisieren, um gemeinsam Bilanz des bisher Erreichten zu ziehen und um die eigenen Arbeiten im internationalen Kreis zu diskutieren. Zwei aktuelle Aspekte des Strahlenschutzes standen im Mittelpunkt der Erörterungen auf dem Symposium.

Zum einen stellte sich die Frage nach den Langzeiteffekten von ionisierenden Strahlungen hoher LET beim Menschen und damit nach quantitativen Daten für eine Risikoabschätzung bei niedrigen Dosen. Hier können die durchgeführten epidemiologischen Studien und experimentellen Untersuchungen zur objektiven Beurteilung des Strahlenrisikos von inkorporierten Radionukliden beitragen, das eines der grundlegenden und kontroversen Probleme in der Diskussion des Kernenergierisikos ist.

Der zweite Aspekt betrifft den Strahlenschutz in der Medizin. Es wurde im Fall der Therapie der ankylosierenden Spondylitis mit ^{224}Ra die Frage nach Nutzen und Risiko dieser therapeutischen Anwendung ionisierender Strahlungen gestellt. Aufgrund der vorgelegten Ergebnisse sollte bei entsprechender Indikationsstellung der therapeutische Erfolg bei weitmöglichster Reduzierung der Strahlenexposition und damit auch der Strahlengefahr erreicht werden.

Beide Fragestellungen sind eng miteinander verknüpft, und es war ein Vorzug dieses Symposiums, dass zu ihrer Beantwortung sowohl klinische Erfahrungen als auch strahlenbiologische Forschungsergebnisse vorgetragen und diskutiert wurden.

H.G. EBERT W.A. MüLLER

On the scientific work of Fritz Schales

My first scientific trip to Germany, in 1966, was largely motivated by a desire to see Fritz Schales, a man I had never met before, but whose paper on the metabolism of radium in man I had studied with keen interest, since I was personally involved in the same problem on the other side of the world.

The interest of Schales in ^{224}Ra metabolism was more than academic, because he, himself, had been injected with ^{224}Ra for the treatment of ankylosing spondylitis, or Morbus Bechterew, as it is usually called in the German-speaking countries. His main interest in ^{224}Ra was its use in therapy, which is the main topic of our present symposium. He was one of the few individuals to have received all 3 of the common forms of treatment (drugs, X-rays, and ^{224}Ra). Based on his own experience, he believed that ^{224}Ra gave the longest-lasting relief with the fewest harmful effects.

As a scientist, he began to convert the historical dosage specifications from elektro-statischen Einheiten (esE) to the presently used µCi of ^{224}Ra (100 esE $\approx$ 14 µCi ^{224}Ra). He was of great help to me personally in my evaluation of the skeletal dose to the Spiess patients. We became lifetime friends.

In 1970, he was asked by Professor Hug to start a new follow-up of over 1000 ^{224}Ra-treated patients that were not included in the patient group investigated by Spiess. The travel involved in this job was very difficult for him, and would have been impossible except for the help of his good wife, who chauffeured him all over Germany. He was particularly concerned about obtaining objective evidence on the benefits of treatment, and with the help of clinical colleagues, developed a detailed examination and questionnaire that has been used before and after ^{224}Ra therapy to evaluate its effect. I was a guest at one of the examinations and was impressed by the urgent need of these patients to be free from pain.

With his own body crippled by ankylosing spondylitis, it was his strong desire to help other spondylitis patients. He very much wished to attend this symposium. In these proceedings you may read his final paper, which he completed only a few days before his untimely death on 3 September 1976.

Charles W. Mays

Opening Address: W. Gössner

Meine Damen und Herren,
Ladies and Gentlemen,

may I welcome you on behalf of the Institute of Biology to this symposium. I thank you all for coming and I am particularly grateful to those who have made a long journey from neighbouring countries or even from overseas. We are fortunate that so many outstanding scientists attend this symposium.

During the next two days we whall have ample opportunity to discuss problems of mutual interest.

May I also thank the Commission of the European Communities, Biology Division and the Gesellschaft für Strahlen- und Umweltforschung for the generous support of this meeting.

Professor Hug who unfortunately can not attend this symposium has asked me to give all of you his best greetings and wishes to a succesful meeting. We all have to pay special tribute to Professor Hug because he has contributed to a great extent to the preparation of this symposium.

May I now give a short introduction into the subject and problems of this symposium. I think that I can be rather brief, because all who are sitting in this room are quite familiar with the subject of this meeting.

The first symposium on the biological effects of ^{224}Ra or Thorium-X was held two years ago at the Alta Lodge in Utah. We all remember a very successful and also enjoyable meeting organized by Professor Mays with a most perfect organization and a homely atmosphere at the same time. A great part of this meeting was in addition devoted to the problems of Thorotrast. The papers and discussions of this symposium have been concentrated on the description and analysis of the late effects specially bone tumors induced by incorporation of these α-emitters and on the problems of dosimetry and radiobiology.

Already during the discussions which we had in preparing this first symposium and again during the Alta-meeting we felt that it would be very important to deal together with clinicians in more detail with the usage of ^{224}Ra in radiotherapy because this treatment of certain diseases of the skeletal system, mainly ankylosing spondylitis has been retained in some clinical centers up to now.

Therefore the main topic of this symposium will be the discussion and analysis of benefit and risk of the therapeutic application of ^{224}Ra in the treatment of ankylosing spondylitis and arthritic diseases.

We all are anxious to learn from the findings and experience of the clinicians and they will certainly also profit from the basic findings of the radiobiologists and experimental pathologists. So I believe that the main purpose of this symposium is to bring these two groups together.

We hope that after these two days we will have a more clear picture about the therapeutic effect of ^{224}Ra in these diseases and also an answer to the question whether this kind of treatment is justified or not.

In the first papers the pathology and clinic of ankylosing spondylitis will be described, a disease of which the aetiology is still unknown and the formal pathogenesis still in discussion. It involves transient and mostly moderate inflammatory changes which are immediately followed by cartilage- and bone-formation. Therefore the analysis of the radiation effects in this disease is closely linked to general problems of the influence of radiation on inflammatory process and bone formation. The latter probably being the more important and based on better clinical and experimental data.

Here I would like to mention the first experimental studies on bone growth in rabbits after incorporation of ^{224}Ra performed by Koch and Spiess in 1951. Since then experimental work on early effects has unfortunately been very much neglected in favour of the late effects studies mainly concerned with the induction of bone tumors.

If we should come tot the conclusion that there may be still a future in ^{224}Ra treatment we certainly will have to do much more experimental work with suitable animal models with spontaneous or experimental induced diseases of the skeletal system.

The very early therapeutic use of ^{224}Ra or Thorium-X already shortly after its discovery by Soddy and Rutherford in 1902 is surprising. There exist about 30 publications already before the first World War dealing with the therapeutic application of Thorium-X in many fields of medicine.

Being a pathologist I would like to mention in this context two fatal accidents after overdosage of Thorium-X which I have found in the old literature.

The first case was a 58 years old female suffering from chronic arthritis. She received 4 injections of Thorium-X and died 8 days after the last injection of 3000 esE. This case was presented by the pathologist Orth during a meeting of the Berlin Medical Society in 1912 (Berl.klin.Wschr. 1912 I, 912).

The second case was published by Hamperl in 1937 (Fig. 1). A young female aged 26 years committed suicide by drinking a solution containing 40.000 esE Thorium-X. She died 14 days later. In both cases the authors have given a very precise autopsy record. Their findings fit completely the picture of a radiation-induced bone marrow syndrome and hemopoetic death.

About 10 years later between 1944 and 1951 the well-known most intensive therapeutic application of ^{224}Ra in form of a combined preparation called Peteosthor has been introduced by Troch (Peteosthor. Neue Wege des Heilens. Verlag Vieweg, Braunschweig, 1949).

After these few historical remarks I finally would like to cite from the text of the protocol of the Berlin Medical Society Meeting in 1912, where the first fatal case has been demonstrated, the following:

'Bei aller berechtigten Betonung der Gefährlichkeit der Thorium-Behandlung möge man übrigens nur nicht das Kind mit dem Bade ausschütten; es gäbe auch therapeutische Effekte des Thorium-X, nicht blosz heftige biologische Wirkungen. Alle starken Mittel sind auch gefährlich.'

I think that this quotation may also be used now 64 years later as motto to this symposium.

Es handelte sich um ein 26jähriges Mädchen, das in selbstmörderischer Absicht 40 000 ESE Thorium X getrunken hatte. Eine nicht näher bestimmbare Menge der Flüssigkeit und damit auch der ESE erbrach sie. Der Krankheitsverlauf ist

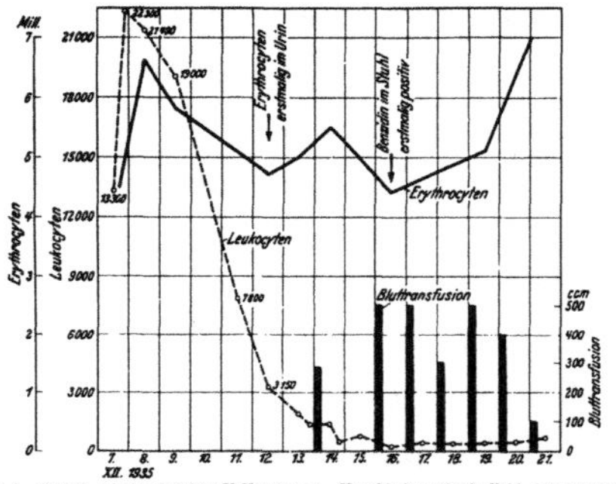

Abb. 1. Fall 1. Akute Thorium-X-Vergiftung. Krankheitsverlauf: Zahl der roten und weißen Blutkörperchen, Bluttransfusionen.

besonders durch das Verhalten des Blutbildes bemerkenswert (s. Abb. 1). Am Tage nach der Einanhme des Giftes war sowohl die Zahl der roten wie weißen Blutkörperchen stark angestiegen. Während sich aber die roten Blutkörperchen, zum Teil wohl auch infolge der vorgenommenen Bluttransfusionen, auf normaler Höhe hielten, ja vor dem am 16. Tage eintretenden Tode noch stark anstiegen, sank die Zahl der weißen Blutkörperchen vom 2. Tage an ständig ab, um am Ende der 1. Woche fast 0 zu erreichen. Diesen Stand behielten die weißen Blutkörperchen trotz aller ärztlichen Maßnahmen bis zum Tode bei. Bei der $1^1/_2$ Stunden nach dem Tode vorgenommenen Leichenöffnung konnte außer einer hämorrhagischen Diathese und starker Parenchymschädigung der Organe eine schwerste pseudomembranös-nekrotisierende Colitis festgestellt werden.

FIGURE 1

Page 378 from H. Hamperl, Akute and chronische, tödliche Strahlenschädigung beim Menschen (2 Fälle), Virchow's Archiv für Pathologische Anatomie und Physiologie und für Klinische Medizin 298, 376-393, 1937.

Zur Klinik der ankylosierenden Spondylitis (Morbus Bechterew)

Professor Dr. P.W. Hartl, Leitender Arzt der Rheumaklinik Landesbad und des Rheumaforschungsinstituts in Aachen

ABSTRACT

The clinical picture of ankylosing spondylitis is described. Actual problems of diagnosis and differential diagnosis are discussed. Modern trends in treating spondylitis patients are pointed out, and modern concepts (indications) on treatment with ^{224}Ra outlined.

Die ankylosierende Spondylitis wird als entzündliche Systemerkrankung des Achsenskeletts, der peripheren Gelenke und verschiedener innerer Organe dem rheumatischen Formenkreis zugeordnet. Sie bevorzugt das männliche Geschlecht und hier wiederum vor allem das jugendliche Alter zwischen dem 15. und 30. Lebensjahr. Die der Erkrankung zugrunde liegenden Entzündungsvorgänge, die nicht nur die Gelenke, sondern auch andere fibrocartilaginöse Strukturen wie Synchondrosen, Bandscheiben, Sehnen- und Ligamentansätze bevorzugen, sind ätiologisch und pathogenetisch bislang nicht ausreichend geklärt. Im Rahmen eines chronisch-progredienten Verlaufes manifestiert sich die ankylosierende Spondylitis klinisch am Achsenskelett unter obligater Beteiligung der Sakroiliakagelenke. In etwa einem Viertel der Fälle, vor allem bei Beginn im jugendlichen Alter, entwickelt sich gleichzeitig eine Polyarthritis. Klinisch stehen der nächtlich verstärkte Rückenschmerz sowie zunehmende Bewegungseinschränkung der

Wirbelsäule im Vordergrund des Krankheitsbildes. Unter den Organmanifestationen der ankylosierenden Spondylitis ist die Uveitis häufig, die Cardiopathie eher selten. Bei der Erkrankung, deren Häufigkeit im europäischen Bereich zwischen 0,08 und 0,2% angegeben wird, führen die zunehmende Versteifung der Wirbelsäule, die Miterkrankung der stammnahen Gelenke, vor allem der Hüften, und in Einzelfällen die Mitbeteiligung innerer Organe (Cardiopathie) zu vorzeitiger Invalidität.

Zur Diagnose führen zunächst die charakteristischen Beschwerden des Patienten, und zwar im Sinne - gelegentlich uncharakteristischer und flüchtiger - lumbaler Rückenschmerzen. Diese sind zunächst lumbal and vor allem in die Kreuzdarmregion lokalisiert, strahlen aber häufig nach cranial hin aus und beziehen die Gesäss- und dorsale Oberschenkelregion (Pseudoischias) sowie die Leistengegend mit ein.

Besonders charakteristisch und für die Differentialdiagnose wichtig, ist die Persistenz des Rückenschmerzes auch nach Ruhigstellung der Wirbelsäule: Der Bechterew-Patient wacht vor Schmerzen meist kurz nach Mitternacht auf und sucht in der Bewegung Schmerzlinderung. Er klagt ferner über eine schmerzhafte Morgensteife des Achsenskeletts, die sich ebenfalls erst nach Bewegung im Verlauf des Tages bessert. Viele Patienten berichten über einen ringförmigen Thoraxschmerz, der erfahrungsgemäss nicht selten als Intercostalneuralgie oder Angina pectoris fehlinterpretiert wird. Sehnenansätze bestimmter Lokalisation wie z.B. am Fersenbein (Kalkaneodynie), in der Sitzbeinregion oder an den Trochanteren sind vielfach spontan oder bei Palpation schmerzhaft.

Bei der klinischen Untersuchung imponiert meist bereits im Frühstadium der Spondilytis als Folge der reflektorischen Verspannung der paravertebralen Rückenmuskulatur eine typische Fehlhaltung unter Aufhebung der physiologischen Lendenwirbellordose. Die Motilität des Achsenskelettes im thorako-lumbalen Übergang der Wirbelsäule ist häufig bereits frühzeitig eingeschränkt, und zwar vor allem für Lateralflexion und Rotation, später dann auch für Vorwärts- und Rückwärtsbeugung. Die für die Erkrankung typischen Ausfälle der Motilität der Wirbelsäule sind schliesslich objektiv messbar. Charakteristisch für die floride Phase des Morbus Bechterew im Initalstadium ist auch die Empfindlichkeit des Iliosakralbereiches bei passiver Stauchung oder bei ruckartig durchgeführter Retroflexion des Hüftgelenkes in Bauch- onder Seitenlage des Kranken (Mennel'scher Handgriff). Im Verlaufe der Erkrankung entwickelt sich eine zunehmende Immobilisierung des gesamten Achsenskeletts, in der Regel von lumbal her nach cranial aufsteigend. Fortgeschrittene Stadien mit weitgehend versteifter Wirbelsäule fallen bereits durch die charakteristische Fehlhaltung - starke Kyphose im thorakalen Bereich ('Pokerrücken') sowie die Zwangshaltung des Kopfes (Protrusio capitis), unter Umständen mit Senkung der Blickachse unter die Horizontale - auf.

Die zunehmende Thoraxstarre wird lange Zeit durch eine vermehrte Bauchatmung kompensiert, die vermehrte Atemarbeit kann aber in Endstadien zu einer respiratorischen Insuffizienz mit der Ausbildung eines chronischen Cor pulmonale führen. Die bei 10 bis 20% der Fälle von ankylosierender Spondylitis auftretende Polyarthritis kann in frühen (präspondylitischen!) Stadien der Erkrankung klinisch-phänomenologisch einem rheumatischen Fieber ähneln. In Spätstadien der ankylosierenden Spondylitis gilt die Arthritis der Hüftgelenke als folgenschwere Komplikation, welche die Prognose auch langfristig gesehen verschlechtert.

Unter den extraartikulären Manifestationen ist die Uveitis als relativ häufige Komplikation zu nennen. Sie tritt in der Regel bilateral rezidivierend auf und ist auch langfristig gesehen prognostisch günstig zu beurteilen. Die Urethritis wird häufig - unter Umständen unter dem Bilde des sogenannten Reitersyndroms und mit einer Balanitis vergesellschaftet - schon in Frühstadien der ankylosierenden Spondylitis beobachtet (und gelegentlich als Gonorrhoe fehlgedeutet!). Bei Mitbeteiligung des Herzens am Krankheitsgeschehen (spondylitische Herzkrankheit) sieht man vor allem elektrokardiographische Veränderungen im Sinne von Überleitungs- und Rhythmusstörungen, eine hämodynamisch relevante Aorteninsuffizienz auf dem Boden der spondylitischen Aortitis ist relativ selten. Das gleiche gilt für Manifestationen im Bereich der Lungen oder neurologische Komplikationen (Cauda equina-Syndrom). Etwa 5 bis 6% aller Fälle mit ankylosierender Spondylitis sind durch eine Amyloidose, in der Regel vom periretikulären Typ kompliziert, an der die Patienten schliesslich unter dem Bilde der Niereninsuffizienz zugrunde gehen.

Als röntgendiagnostische Leitsymptome der Bechterew'schen Erkrankung gelten einmal die bilaterale Sakroiliitis in ihren verschiedenen röntgenphänomenologischen Varianten sowie als Beweis für die Spondylitis die vor allem in fortgeschrittenen Stadien ausgebildeten Syndesmophyten. In frühen, röntgenologisch noch latenten Fällen kann der szintigraphische Nachweis der Kreuzdarmbein-Gelenkarthritis diagnostisch weiterführen.

Im labormedizinischen Bereich sind krankheitstypische serologische Befunde wie z.B. beim rheumatischen Fieber, der rheumatoiden Arthritis oder beim Lupus erythematodes für die ankylosierende Spondylitis bisher nicht bekannt. Neuerdings findet aber die klinische Diagnose durch Nachweis des Histokompatibilitätsantigens HLA B 27 eine wesentliche Stütze, das bei dieser Krankheit in mehr als 95% der Fälle gefunden wird. Die Krankheitsaktivität wird anhand der klassischen 'Entzündungsparameter' beurteilt, wie Blutsenkungsgeschwindigkeit, Serum-Elektrophorese sowie Serumspiegel von Haptoglobin, Ceruplasmin und Alpha-1-saurem Glykoprotein ohne dass in jedem Falle eine strenge Beziehung zu den klinischen Aktivitäten bestehen muss. Pathologische Laborparameter, die keinen direkten Bezug zur ankylosierenden Spondylitis haben und auf eine Affektion innerer Organe hinweisen, müssen stets an die Möglichkeit von Therapieschäden oder an das Vorliegen einer Amyloidose denken lassen.

Eine kausale *Therapie* der ankylosierenden Spondylitis ist bisher nicht möglich. Im Hinblick auf diese Situation wird man im Rahmen therapeutischer Überlegungen vor allem eine möglichst optimale Erhaltung der Motilität des Achsenskeletts sowie die Prävention folgenschwerer Deformationen des Achsenskeletts im Auge haben.

Die gezielte Bewegungstherapie des Achsenskeletts und betroffener peripherer Gelenke sowie krankengymnastische Massnahmen zur Erhaltung der Atemfunktion sind die Basis eines langfristig angelegten Behandlungsprogrammes. Dieses wird durch eine sinnvoll an die bestehenden Motilitätseinschränkungen abgestimmte beschäftigungstherapeutische Behandlung ergänzt.

Medikamentös hat sich gegen den Rückenschmerz die Gabe von 3 x 50 mg Indometacin/Tag, ergänzt durch ein Suppositorium à 100 mg für die Nacht, bewährt. Bei Unverträglichkeit - Schwindel, Nausea, Konzentrationsschwäche - kann man auf Phenylbutazon oder ein neueres, nicht steroidales Antirheumatikum zurückgreifen unter strikter Beachtung möglicher Therapienebenwirkungen. Glucocorticosteroide haben bei der Behandlung der ankylosierenden Spondylitis enttäuscht. Eine vorübergehende Anwendung ist bei der Uveitis (möglichst lokal) angezeigt. Eine Therapie mit Röntgenstrahlen oder intravenöser Injektion von Radionukliden ist trotz des unbestrittenen guten analgetischen Effektes wegen der Gefahr von Nebenwirkungen heute nicht mehr generell zu empfehlen. Diese Therapieformen sollten auf stark progredient verlaufende Fälle beschränkt bleiben, bei denen die medikamentöse Therapie analgetisch nicht ausreicht oder wegen bestehender Kontraindikation (peptisches Magen-Darm-Ulcus) nicht möglich ist. Nutzen und Risiken einer solchen Behandlung müssen sorgsam abgewogen und mit dem Patienten besprochen werden.

Die chirurgische Behandlung der ankylosierenden Spondylitis hat vor allem durch die Arthroplastik der Hüftgelenke einen wesentlichen Fortschritt gebracht, da sie Patienten in fortgeschrittenen Stadien wieder gehfähig machen kann. Die Columnotomie, die den Oberkörper des Patienten durch Osteotomie und Rückwärtsneigung der Wirbelsäule um 25 bis 45% aufrichtet, kann vor allem wegen der Hebung der Blickachse für den Kranken segensreich sein. Wegen der noch bestehenden Operationsrisiken ist dieser Eingriff aber sicher nur in besonders gelagerten, sehr fortgeschrittenen Fällen angezeigt.

Die Therapie der ankylosierenden Spondylitis ist um so effektiver, je frühzeitiger die Diagnose gestellt wird.

Erfahrungsgemäss wird die Erkrankung aber im Frühstadium, das heisst innerhalb der ersten 3 Jahre nach Beschwerdebeginn meist nicht erkannt. Häufige Fehldiagnosen sind: 'Morbus Scheuermann, Diskopathien (Operation!), Weichteilrheumatismus, psychogene Beschwerden'. Vor allem bei Frauen, bei denen die Erkrankung oft milde und vielfach ohne starke Progression verläuft, wird der Morbus Bechterew häufig viel zu spät diagnostiziert. Beim Jugendlichen, bei dem die Erkrankung der peripheren Gelenke der Spondylitis vorausgehen kann, wird unter der Diagnose 'seronegative-Polyarthritis' erfahrungsgemäss nicht selten ein betroffenes Einzelgelenk ruhig gestellt mit dem Ergebnis einer rasch eintretenden Ankylose und Gelenkversteifung.

An eine ankylosierende Spondylitis sollte der Arzt differentialdiagnostisch immer dann denken,

wenn *lumbalgiforme Rückenschmerzen*

nachts persistieren,

auf Indometacin oder Phenylbutazon prompt und nachhaltig ansprechen,

mit einer Bewegungseinschränkung vor allem im Lendenwirbelsäulenbereich verbunden sind,

mit Thoraxschmerzen einhergehen,

mit Schmerzen an Sehnenansätzen (Kalkaneodynie) kombiniert sind,

mit einer Uveitis einhergehen,

im Anschluss an einen Morbus Reiter oder

zusammen mit einer entzündlichen Erkrankung des Darmes auftreten (enteropathische Spondylitis),

einen männlichen Jugendlichen betreffen sowie

mit einer erhöhten Blutsenkung verbunden sind.

Mit dem röntgenologischen Nachweis der bilateralen Sakroiliitis ist die Diagnose der ankylosierende Spondylitis auch in Frühphasen der Erkrankung in der Regel rasch und sicher zu stellen. In röntgenologisch zweifelhaften Fällen hilft die Szintigraphie oder ggf. die Bestimmung des HLA B 27-Antigens weiter.

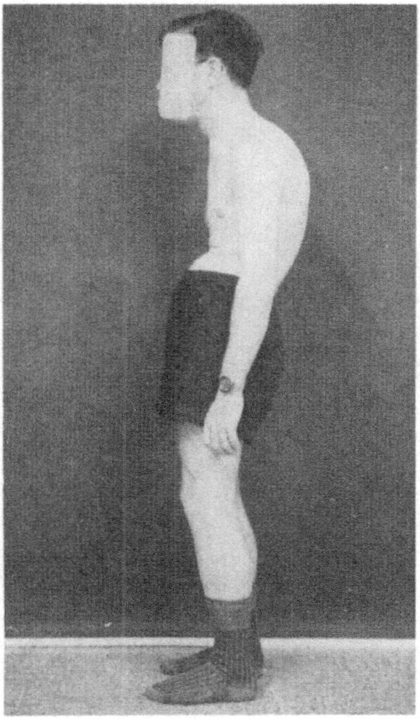

FIGURE 1

Typische Körperhaltung bei fortgeschrittenem Morbus Bechterew.

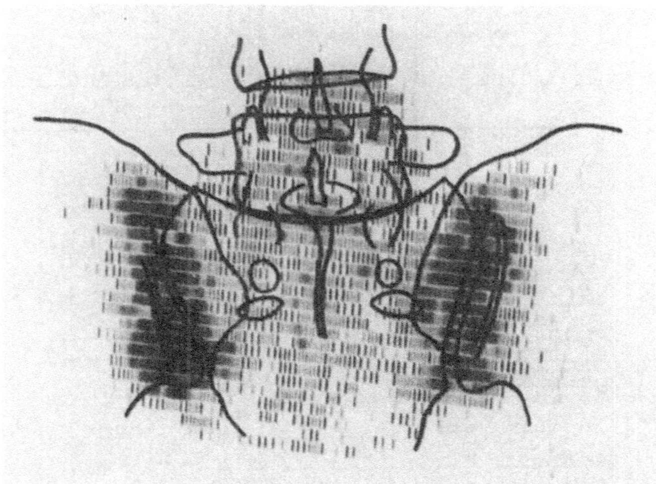

FIGURE 2

Szintigrafischer Befund im Frühstadium eines Morbus Bechterew (floride Kreuzdarmbein-Gelenkarthritis).

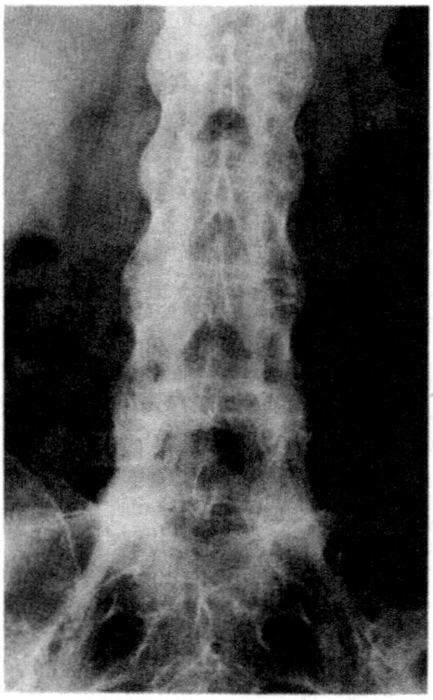

FIGURE 3

Röntgenbild der Wirbelsäule im Spätstadium des Morbus Bechterew ('Bambusstab').

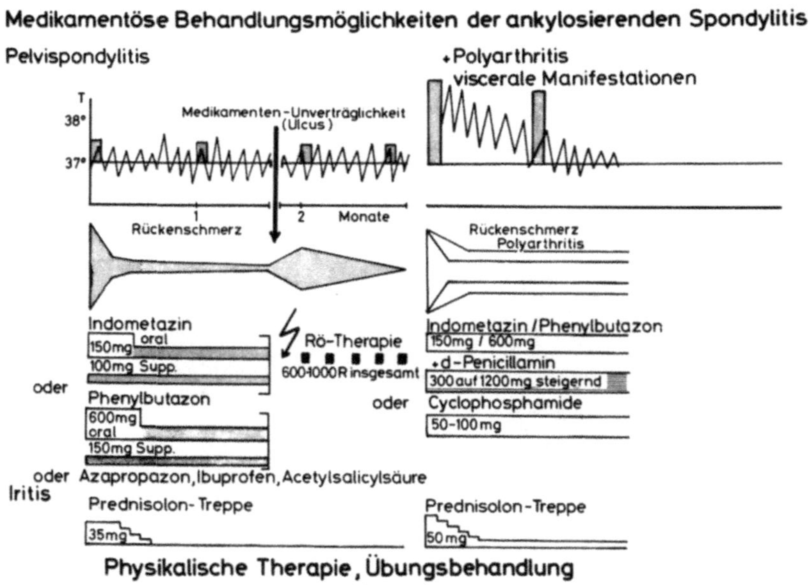

FIGURE 4

Übersicht über medikamentöse Behandlungsmöglichkeiten bei ankylosierender Spondylitis.

Pathology and radiology of ankylosing spondylitis

Professor Dr.med. F. Schilling, Zentrum für Rheuma-Pathologie
6500 Mainz, Rheinstrasse 4, Federal Republic of Germany

ABSTRACT

1. The study presented is based on a clinical and roentgeno-morphological investigation of 2000 patients with ankylosing spondylitis. A statistical analysis, and in some cases a pathological investigation, was done on 600 patients.
2. Within the study a profile is provided of:
   a. the early stages of the disease,
   b. abortive forms,
   c. special forms and variants of the ailment such as: juvenile ankylosing spondylitis, psoriatic spondylitis and chronic Reiter's syndrome.
3. The ambiguous nature of ankylosing spondylitis is described with its partly inflammatory spondylarthritic, partly metaplastic ossifying components.
4. The transformation of bone in border-line regions to the connective tissue is recognized as the principle of the underlying process. It finds its realization in the models of the inflammatory ossifying fibro-ostitis of insertions and the disco-vertebral destruction. The enthesopathy represents the morphological bridge to the psoriatic-arthritic and spondylitic syndrome and to the chronic Reiter's syndrome.
4. A statistical analysis involving 600 patients was done on arthritides of the joints of the extremities. This arthritis has been shown to be a nosological component of the ailment.

5. In ankylosing spondylitis, the patient's age at the oneset of the disease is a decisive factor in the type of manifestation *(nosomorphosis)*:
   a. in the juvenile form the arthritis of the lower extremities is dominant; the juvenile state is predisposed to the spondylarthritic type;
   b. the metaplastic ossification of the vertebral column is the increasingly characteristic feature of the disease after the age of twenty years; the aging state is predisposed to the syndesmophytic type.
6. The study of morphology, topography and pathogenesis of the syndesmophytes show ossification at three levels:
   a. the anulus-type (classical and most frequent type),
   b. the sub-ligamentous type,
   c. the ligamentous type (rare, morphologically related to hyperostotic ankylosing spondylosis).
7. The segment of mobility, supported and ankylosed by syndesmophytes, is subjected to new static conditions and to other formative laws causing a transformation of the vertebral body with a productive and a resorptive component. The destructive phase of this process takes place as marginal spondylitis, anterior spondylitis, discitis and spondylodiscitis.
   The knowledge of mechanical strain explains the alteration of the vertebral body in terms of structural dynamics; the change of functional dynamics within the stiffening process of ankylosing spondylitis creates the 'strain-dynamical' prerequisites for the morphological variability of spondylitis in this malady. Therefore, the destructive phase of spondylitis is the manifestation of a structural osseous transformation of the vertebral body dependent on statics and function.
8. The results obtained are summarized and evaluated for clinical differential diagnosis.

Indication for ^{224}Ra-therapy in ankylosing spondylitis (Morbus Struempell-Bechterew-Marie)

Professor Dr.med. W. Koch, Professor of the Orthopaedic Clinic of the University Münster/Westfalen, Federal Republic of Germany

SUMMARY

^{224}Ra therapy in ankylosing spondylitis has been employed successfully at our hospital since 1948, administering 10 i.v. injections à 28 μCi at weekly intervals. However, the treatment is only indicated in phase II and III of the disease when therapeutic resistance of the painfully inflamed vertebral and iliosacral joints is observed and progressive spine stiffening is established roentgenographically. It is not allowed in the initial phase when only the iliosacral joints are involved as iliosacral arthritis, nor in the last phase when spine stiffening with or without involvement of the joints at the extremities is complete.

Due to the antiosteoblastic effect of the alpha-radiation of ^{224}Ra and the antiphlogistic effect of the beta- and gamma-radiation emitted by its disintegration products, the disease is favourably influenced during phase II and III so that active therapeutic exercises as well as balneological treatment becomes possible while the patient is hospitalized for 10 weeks.

INTRODUCTION

In the German medical literature the term 'spondylarthritis ankylopoetica' (Fraenkel 1903) is generally used to define the inflammatory stiffening of the vertebral column. It emphasizes the initial inflammation process in the posterior vertebral and costovertebral joints. The term 'ankylosing spondylitis' (a.sp.) generally used in the Anglo-American literature is derived from 'spondylitis ankylopoetica', as introduced by Simmonds (1903) to emphasize the less frequent start of the disease as so-called Bechterew-discitis (Diehlmann 1966).

The clinical cases published at the end of the 19th century have already demonstrated that the etiology of the disease is uncertain. Thus Struempell (1884) described the painless ascending osseous stiffening of the spine, while Bechterew (1893) mentioned the painful ankylosis in kyphotic attitude, and Pierre-Marie (1998) pointed out the additional involvement of hip and shoulder joints.

Evaluating the experiences of the past 25 years in pathological anatomy and clinical roentgenology, a distinction between 3 different manifestations seems possible and useful for therapeutic purposes:

1. The purely osseous form of a.sp. with more or less painless stiffening of the spine,
2. the inflammatory rheumatic disease of the spine which is very painful, and
3. the mixed form where the painful inflammatory attacks alternate with periods of painless, bland, osseous stiffening.

In all cases it may come to a remission, to osteoporosis of the axial skeleton, and to an osseous or inflammatory affliction of the proximal and peripheral joints.

Of the 774 patients with a.sp. treated at our hospital, we saw the purely osseous form in 155 cases and the rheumatic form in 57 cases. Most patients, i.e. 542, had the so-called mixed form.

Until 25 years ago, the treatment of a.sp. was only symptomatic and quite often polypragmatic. Only in the past 25 years a causal therapy has been developed according to the different manifestations of the disease cited above. Thus, for the purely inflammatory form as well as for the mixed form of a.sp. antirheumatic drugs are used, while corticosteroids are forbidden because the disease itself already causes osteoperosis which would only be intensified by the application of corticosteroids. If antiphlogistics and analgesics are not or no longer effective, radiotherapy with ^{224}Ra is indicated when the roentgenogram displays onset or increase of ossification zones with formation of syndesmophytes between the thoracic and the lumbar spine, or osseous fusion of the sacro-iliac and the small vertebral joints (phase II and III). The object of this therapy - which should be administered only very critically - is to interrupt the ossification process in the axial skeleton, at the same time inhibiting the painful inflammation in the small vertebral joints. An already existing ossification cannot be reversed by this therapy.

RADIATION EFFECTS ON BONE TISSUE

Animal experiments and clinical observation permitted a better understanding of the effects of corpuscular alpha- and beta-radiation of ^{224}Ra on bone tissue and made an effective radiotherapy of a.sp. possible (Koch 1957). Experiments with ^{224}Ra on rabbits and also on man led to some important conclusions concerning the ^{224}Ra emission, dispersion, and radiation effects on ossification.

^{224}Ra is a calcium homologue. It is taken up almost exclusively by osseous tissue where it combines with the bone salt in physiological as well as pathological calcifications. The primary trabeculae of the epiphyseal cartilage and the fracture callus absorb the highest amount of ^{224}Ra (see Fig. 1).

The dosage which we use parenterally interrupts the enchondral ossification in the epiphyseal cartilage and in the fracture callus. The radiation-induced osteopathy of the metaphysis is exclusively caused by the damage inflicted on the bone cells and signals the disturbed process of enchondral ossification. The radiation effects on the

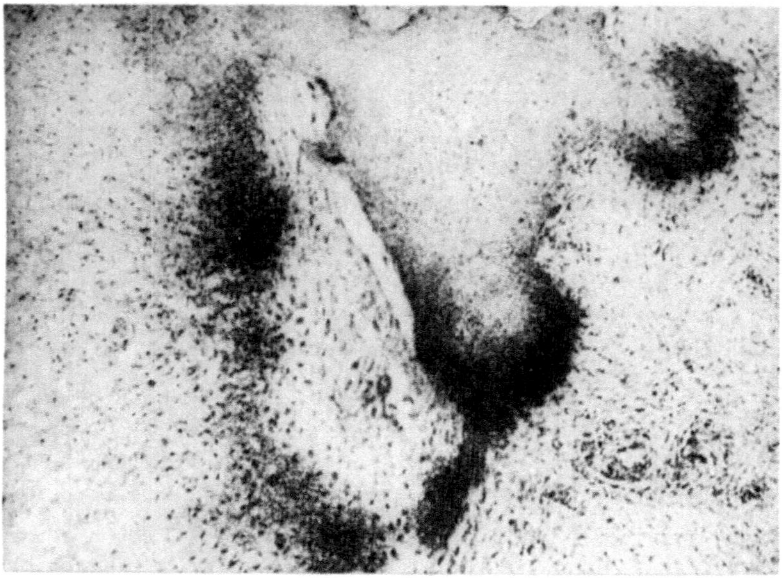

FIGURE 1

Autoradiography of a 4-week old fracture callus of a rabbit. Peripheral ^{224}Ra deposits into primitive trabeculae and caldividation of vesicular cartilage (left).

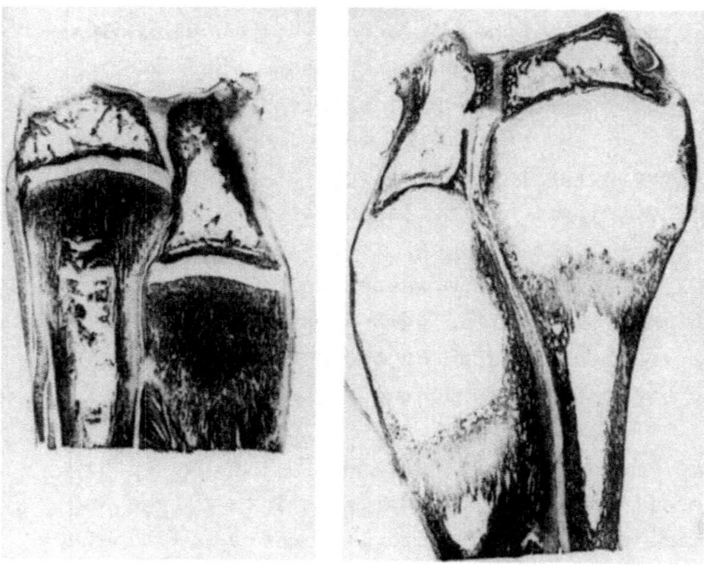

FIGURE 2

Normal (left) and distorted distal ulnar-radial ossification zones (right) of 10-week old rabbit after 6 weeks of ^{224}Ra treatment.

epiphyseal cartilage (see Fig. 2) and the fracture callus account for the observed delay of growth in height and for the delayed or even inhibited fracture healing in man and animal (see Fig. 3).

CLINICAL EXPERIENCE WITH ^{224}RA

Clinical experience with ^{224}Ra for the treatment in a.sp. were gained several decades before the basic research results mentioned above were published. We introduced the therapy of a.sp. with ^{224}Ra at our hospital in 1948 with weekly injections of 28 µCi up to a total of 10 injections.

While the primary and enchondral pathological ossification is disturbed at an early stage by alpha-emitters from the accumulated ^{224}Ra in the calciferous and bradytroph tissue of the spine, the inflammatory changes in the small vertebral joints as well as in the paraosseous tissue are inhibited by far-reaching beta- and gamma-emitters.

In some cases of a.sp. the patients suffer severe pain during the first 24 hours after the ^{224}Ra injection. After 10 injections, or in some cases already after 5 injections, there is analgia. Analgia must not be enforced by increasing the total number of injections above 10. Encouraged by the good results (Pitzen 1949), the method of ^{224}Ra therapy in a.sp. has been adopted by several other (mostly orthopaedic) university hospitals in Germany, and a large number of publications has appeared since reporting good or even excellent results with this therapy.

The encouraging subjective statements of the patients regarding pain relief in the spine and joints can be objectivated by testing the flexibility of the vertebral column and of the affected joints. Further information on the course of the disease and an explanation for the analgia is gained by the blood sedimentation rate (BSR). Normalization or at least slackening of the blood sedimentation rate was found in 66 per cent of our cases, supporting the roentgenographic findings and statements of disappearance

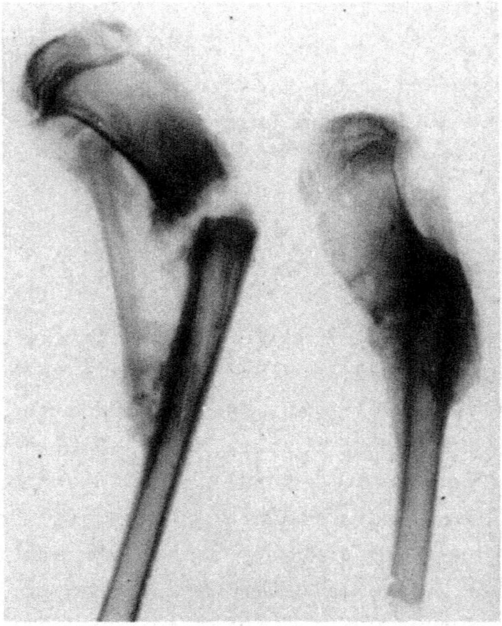

FIGURE 3

Osteotomy of a rabbit tibia. After ^{224}Ra no fracture healing. After ^{32}P normal callus (right).

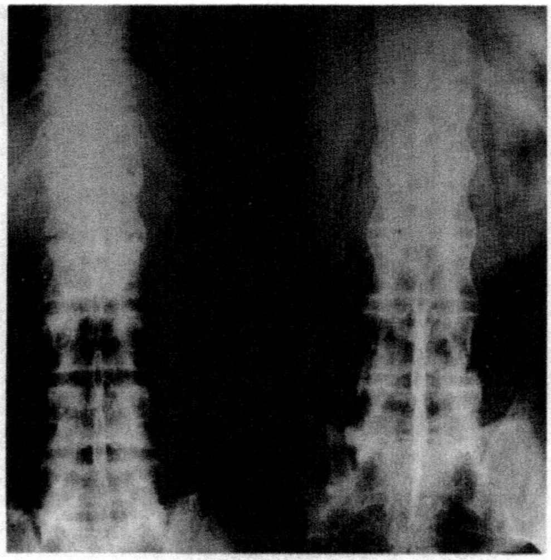

FIGURE 4

71-year old man, bamboo spine, before (left) and 10 years after ^{224}Ra treatment (right).

of pain. In 12 per cent of all cases the blood sedimentation rate was increased due to osteoporosis or to a partly persistent inflammatory process; in 24 per cent of our cases a relapse occurrence of iritis may have been responsible for the increased blood sedimentation rate.

Regarding the return-to-work quota of our patients, we can say that more than 50 per cent were able to take up their previous work. Only 14 per cent had to change it and find a physically less strenuous type of work.

Roentgenographic evaluation of the spine and of the main joints showed that - with an exception of the purely or predominantly inflammatory cases - in spite of ^{224}Ra therapy the ossification process of the spine continued during the 10 to 20 years following the injections. The joints, however, remained almost unaffected. This painless osseous stiffening of the axial skeleton occurred mainly in the purely osseous-inflammatory type of a.sp. It did not prompt us to repeat the ^{224}Ra therapy. As yet it is uncertain whether the therapy with ^{224}Ra is responsible for the absence or discontinuation of spine stiffening seen in some patients.

The following examples representing the three types of a.sp. may help to elucidate the aforesaid. First, there is the case of a 71-year old man as an example for the purely osseous type of a.sp. His lumbar and thoracic spine stiffened painlessly to the shape of a bamboo rod during the 10 years following ^{224}Ra therapy with 350 μCi (see Fig. 4). The cervical spine remained mobile.

The inflammatory osseous type of a.sp. is represented by the case of a 43-year old physician where the ossification of the spine was arrested during the 17 years following the injection of 280 μCi of ^{224}Ra. The roentgenogram of the lumbar spine and of the sacral region shows incomplete fusion of both sacro-iliac sutures. The vertebral joints are not fused. The onset of syndesmophyte formation in the lumbar spine is delayed (see Fig. 5.).

An example form the mixed of a.sp. is the case of a 46-year old patient where the ossification process at the hip joint was arrested after an endoprosthetic operation and post-

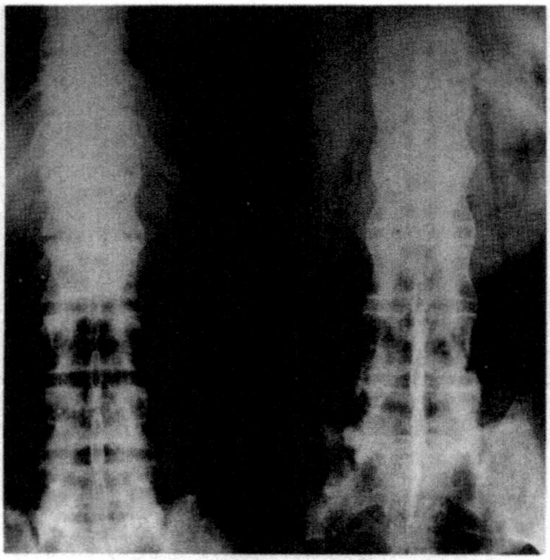

FIGURE 5

43-year old man. After ^{224}Ra treatment no discernible ossification, hardly any syndesmophyte formation from 1951 (left) to 1968 (right).

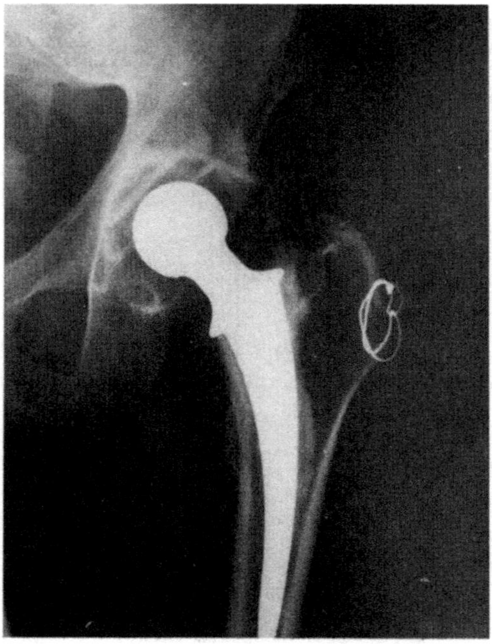

FIGURE 6

No ossification of hip joint after endoprostetic operation and postoperative ^{224}Ra treatment in 46-year old man.

operative ^{224}Ra treatment with weekly injections of 28 μCi each for 10 weeks.

Intensive physiotherapy consisting mainly of respiratory exercises, swimming, gymnastics, etc. should be performed once analgia has been reached. The patient should also learn spine straightening exercises and practice mobilization of the joints.

It is justified to question the value of the treatment with radio-active substances. They should be applied very carefully and only if no other effective treatment of the disease is possible. Regarding the contraindications, the ^{224}Ra therapy must not be administered in adolescents, during pregnancy, nor in patients with impaired parenchymatous and blood-forming organs and lung tuberculosis. With this in mind and adhering to a dosage of 10 injections of 28 μCi no immediate or late impairments are to be expected. Leukopenia, agranulocytosis, panmyelophthisis or leukaemia have not been observed so far, neither have there been any reports regarding ill effects on the male or female gonads after i.v. ^{224}Ra therapy. To our knowledge the children of those patients who received ^{224}Ra treatment are also normal. Our present state of knowledge is not sufficient to decide whether gene mutation is induced by radiation, therefore we recommend family planning before ^{224}Ra therapy is started. It must be remembered, though, that the disposition for a.sp. is hereditary.

A malignant bone tumor has not been observed in any of our 695 a.sp. patients. All of them were followed up clinically and roentgenographically, some of them for as long as 28 years.

Summarizing we can say that the value of the ^{224}Ra therapy in conjunction with active therapeutic exercises has been fully acknowledged, presupposing careful consideration of the indication and contraindication. As such it is a real adjunct in the hands of an experienced physician and will probably reach an important position as therapeutic means in the treatment of a.sp.

Literature on request from the author.

Problems and results of a new follow-up study – ^{224}Ra in adult ankylosing spondylitis patients*

F. Schales †, Institut für Biologie Gesellschaft für Strahlen- und Umweltforschung mbH, D-6000 Frankfurt, Paul-Ehrlich-Str. 15 u. 20, Federal Republic of Germany

ABSTRACT

Methods applied in these epidemiological studies are explained (questionnaires, personal contacts, clinical investigations and re-investigations).

The causes of death of deceased patients were listed and compared with those of the normal population.

In the last few decades several follow-up studies on late radiation effects have been started. From these may be mentioned two examples:

a. The follow-up of ankylosing spondylitis patients treated in England with X-rays (1). Sir Brian Windeyer will give us in his paper some additional information (2).
b. Persons injected with the ^{232}Th-containing X-ray contrast medium 'Thorotrast' are followed up in several countries. These problems together with those of the Thorium daughter product ^{224}Ra have been treated also in the first ^{224}Ra-Symposium in Alta, Utah 1974 (3).

The main problem in all of these studies is an exact radiation dosimetry. Without the knowledge of radiation dose we cannot postulate realistic dose-effect relations.

* In association with EURATOM (Contract No. 090-72-1 BIO D).

At the first symposium 2 years ago it was reported on dosimetric work done for the ^{224}Ra studies (4). We had decided to calculate as a first step the 'average skeletal dose' i.e. the absorbed radiation energy from ^{224}Ra and its daughters formed in situ, divided by the mass of the whole skeleton. Thus we assume that ^{224}Ra be uniformly distributed throughout the whole skeleton. Due to the short half-life of 3.62 days this is surely not correct, but it gave us the possibility of a direct comparison with the ^{226}Ra study. A more realistic dose can be calculated by multiplying this dose by a factor taking into account the penetration of ^{224}Ra into a bone layer of a few microns. This problem will be discussed certainly at this symposium.

The general equation for the conversion of the administered amount of ^{224}Ra in μCi into rad units was proposed by Spiess and Mays (5) as 1 μCi = 0.2 rad - for adults (70 kg body weight).

Some short remarks to the history of ^{224}Ra treatment in Germany: More than 30 years ago Troch (6) believed to have found a remedy especially for bone and joint tuberculosis by combining ^{224}Ra with platinum and eosin. He was unable to see that his 'Peteosthor' was ineffective in tuberculosis treatment, even after prolonging again and again the treatment, thus increasing the administered doses with the horrible consequences as detected later on life. On the other hand he did not perceive that he had found by chance an effective remedy for the treatment of ankylosing spondylitis. In accordance with the proposal of Koch (7), the dose was drastically reduced to 10-12 injections of 28 μCi, omitting Pt and eosin as of January, 1950.

Up to now Koch has treated in his hospital in Münster 890 patients and has surveyed the success of this method (7). Spiess et al. (8) observed an enormous increase of bone lesions among ^{224}Ra-treated patients of the Troch hospital. He began to locate as many patients as possible, but as this hospital does no longer exist, (and for other reasons) he could contact only about 50% of the patients, the fate of the rest remains unknown.

In the first treatment period most of the patients had received doses of several hundreds or even thousands of rads, the low-dose group being rather small.

As it turned out to be necessary to know more about the effects of doses below 100 rads, a follow-up study of the ankylosing spondylitis patients as mentioned above was started 1971 in the GSF (in association with EURATOM). Most of the doses were between 50-60 rads.

In the meantime 1850 of the names of ankylosing spondylitis patients could be found out in 10 hospitals (including the cases located by Spiess), and as only 1 or 2 greater hospitals could not yet be contacted, I hope to have found out the bulk of the patients available in Germany.

It is a problem and one has to apply different strategies to find out the names of patients who had been treated up to 25 years ago. Most of the difficulties arose when the patient in question had died in the meantime. The Health Offices were in no way willing to give information due to the fear to hurt the private sphere of a patient. With the help of relatives, family doctors and hospitals most causes of death could be found out, but up to 10 letters were necessary per patient.

One aspect must be stated here. Contrary to many other diseases the patients suffering from ankylosing spondylitis are in the majority of cases willing to cooperate, especially if one can convince them that their information will help to improve the treatment method and to make available the experiences to other patients.

In the course of my data collecting I observed that numerous patients had doses of more than 90 rad (a 'critical dose', see later). This was due partly to the fact that in some hospitals the treatment had been repeated. Moreover I had found out several patients treated with Peteosthor in the Troch manner.

On the other hand Spiess had in his low-dose group 158 ankylosing spondylitis patients. Moreover the 4 sarcoma cases with the lowest doses (90 rad, 106 rad, 129 rad, 207 rad) were all ankylosing spondylitis patients.

In the following tables preliminary results of my study are given. They are based on a first computer display which still contains several mistakes. But the final results will not differ for more than 1-2% from these values.

Table 1 gives a survey of patient contacts. More than 1100 patients could be contacted directly, by questionnaire, but also by personal contact or a repeated hospital confinement. About 250 among them have been or are being re-investigated clinically. Another 156 patients have not yet been contacted as they had been ^{224}Ra-treated only 2-4 years ago. 418 Patients have died in the meantime. About 150 addresses could not be found out, so that these patients (about 8%) are lost for the follow-up.

Table 2: About 1625 patients with known radiation doses (included the Spiess patients) are grouped as follows. 1256 (Spiess 158) had doses below 90 rad, the group of 50-59 rad alone 571, the neighboring groups 192 and 214, respectively 369 patients (Spiess 225) had doses higher than 90 rad.

Table 3 gives a survey of the causes of death. In 32 cases the cause of death could not be found out, but 14 of them died 5 years after ^{224}Ra-treatment so that they are lost to the follow-up if we lock for late radiation damages. - The 59 neoplasms among 418 deaths (14%) are lower than in the normal population (20%). 4 Osteosarcoma cases are those of the Spiess series. 2 Patiens died from panmyelopathia,

TABLE I

CONTACTS WITH ANKYLOSING SPONDYLITIS PATIENTS (END OF 1975)

Kind of contact	Sum of patients	Per cent
Unknown, no contact	148	8
Deaths	418	23
Personal contact	1101	60
Not yet contacted 5 years	156	8.5
	1823	99.5

250 Patients were clinically re-investigated

TABLE II

DOSE DISTRIBUTION GROUPS

Dose region (rad)	All patients	Spiess patients
< 39	160	35
40-49	192	10
50-59	571	45
60-69	214	48
70-79	75	14
80-89	44	6
> 90	369	225
	1625	383

Additional informations:

Female/male = 192/1429 = 1 : 7.5
Peteosthor 331 patients

TABLE III

DEATH CAUSES OF ^{224}RA-TREATED PATIENTS
WITH ANKYLOSING SPONDYLITIS

Number of patients	Death cause	Per cent	
56	heart infarction	13.4	29
65	other heart and circulation diseases	15.6	
59	neoplasias	14.1	
39	accidents, suicides	9.3	
32	decline of life	7.6	
30	respiratory tract	7.2	
19	kidney	4.6	
18	cachexia	4.3	
10	tuberculosis	2.4	
58	other diseases	13.9	
32 (18 + 14)	unknown	7.6	
418		100.00	

one of them 20 years after 450 rad Peteosthor and additional X-raying. The second died 4 years after 54 rad Peteosthor but he had abused pyrazolone drugs and worked with aniline paints. 2 Other cases have to be mentioned here although the connection with radiation is improbable: a case of reticulosis of the bone marrow and the other from paraproteinaemic anaemia. - The bulk of the patients died from heart diseases (29%) including 13.4% heart infarcts.

The results of the clinical re-investigations which included the search for late radiation effects will be given in a following paper by Schmitt. (9)

Genetic damages seem to be improbable. Among 69 children born after ^{224}Ra-therapy of one of the parents only one case of an eye defect was observed.

REFERENCES

1. Sharp, J. and E.C. Easson, Deep X-ray therapy in spondylitis. Brit.Med.J. I, 619-623 (1954).
2. Windeyer, B., X-ray therapy in the treatment of ankylosing spondylitis. This symposium.
3. International Symposium on 'Biological Effects of Injected ^{224}Ra and Thorotrast'. Health Physics, in press.
4. Schales, F., Brief history of ^{224}Ra-usage in radiotherapy and radiobiology. Health Physics, in press.
5. Spiess, H. and C.W. Mays, Bone cancers induced by ^{224}Ra (Th X) in children and adults. Health Physics 19, 713-729 (1970).
6. Troch, P., Peteosthor - Neue Wege des Heilens. Vieweg & Sohn, Braunschweig, 1949.
7. Koch, W., Ergebnisse einer zwanzigjährigen parenteralen Thorium-X-Therapie der knöchern-entzündlichen Wirbelsäulenversteifung (Morbus Bechterew). Verh.Dtsch.Ges. Rheumatol. 1, 132-140 (1969).
8. Spiess, H., Poppe, H. and H. Schoen, Strahlen-induzierte Knochentumoren nach Thorium-X-Behandlung. Monatsschrift für Kinderheilkunde 110, 198-201 (1962).

9. Schmitt, E., Therapeutical results in a follow-up study on ^{224}Ra therapy of ankylosing spondylitis. This symposium.

Addendum to the previous paper: risk to bone from present ^{224}Ra therapy

Charles W. Mays, Radiobiology Laboratory, University of Utah Medical Center, Salt Lake City, Utah, USA 84132
(Supported by USERDA Contract EY-76-C-02-0119)

ABSTRACT

Present ^{224}Ra treatment for ankylosing spondylitis in Germany consists of 10 weekly intravenous injections, each of 28 μCi ^{224}Ra, giving a cumulative dose of about 56 rad to the marrow-free skeleton of a reference 70-kg man. Among the ^{224}Ra patients followed by Professor Heinz Spiess (mostly at high doses), 54 cases of bone sarcoma have occurred, but none below 90 rad. Dr. Fritz Schales ascertained the health status of about 1170 ankylosing spondylitis patients with skeletal doses from ^{224}Ra below 90 rad (mean ∿ 56 rad). The average follow up time of these patients was about 12 years.
Dr. Schales found 1 case of reticulum cell sarcoma of bone marrow, at an average skeletal dose between 60 and 112 rad. The bone sarcoma risk throughout lifetime, following present ^{224}Ra treatment, is calculated to be between lower and upper limits (P = 0.05) of 0 and 0.6% if one skeletal sarcoma has occurred in the 1170 patients below 90 rad, or between 0 and 0.4%, if no sarcomas have occurred. No assessment has been made of the possible risk from other effects, such as kidney diseases, liver diseases, and cataracts.

INTRODUCTION

Dr. Fritz Schales (1) had hoped to evaluate the bone sarcoma risk associated with the present ^{224}Ra therapy now used in Germany (10 weekly injections, totalling 280 μCi ^{224}Ra, giving a calculated average skeletal dose of about 56 rads to the 70-kg marrow-free skeleton of reference man). But his deteriorating health allowed him to assemble only 'the naked data' before his untimely death on 3 September 1976. In this paper, I will use the available information to make the analysis that my friend was unable to complete. In no way does this obviate the need to improve the evaluation as new data become available. It is my sincere hope that the follow up of these patients will continue.

POPULATION AT RISK

Table 1 of Schales (1) indicates that by the end of 1975 he had obtained the health status of 1519 adult spondylitis patients treated with ^{224}Ra (1101 alive and 418 dead), which included 383 spondylitis patients from the Spiess series. His Table 2 shows that for the combined traced and untraced patients of known dose, about 77% had average skeletal doses below 90 rad (mean ∿ 56 rad). Thus, the number of traced spondylitic patients below 90 rad was about (0.77)(1519) = *1170 patients*. (The 90 rad dose is of interest because it is the lowest dose at which a bone sarcoma has developed in the Spiess patients (2, 3)).

During his presentation, on 14 April 1975, at the EULEP (European Late Effects Project) meeting in Brussels, Dr. Schales reported an average follow up time of 11 years. Presumably, as of his data cutoff (December 1975), his average follow up was about *12 years*.

A RETICULUM CELL SARCOMA OF BONE MARROW

Dr. Schales wrote me, that he had found a case of reticulum cell sarcoma of bone marrow. (4) Because it was the only known case of skeletal sarcoma among the patients that he had traced personally, it will be described in some detail.

The male patient, MaF (Schales patient number 587), born on 27 November 1907, was given 12 weekly injections, totalling 2400 esE (336 μCi ^{224}Ra), at Münster in 1954, for the treatment of ankylosing spondylitis. On 5 July 1970, the patient died with a histologically diagnosed reticulum cell sarcoma of bone marrow. This tumor involved the sternum humerus, and vertebrae. Extramedullary hematopoiesis was observed in the spleen. Widespread tumor infiltrate was found in the spleen and liver. Remarkable was the finding that the lymph nodes were not enlarged.

Normally, the weight of the marrow-free skeleton is taken as 10% of body weight, (5) a procedure which seems reasonable, except for persons who are unusually fat or thin. The recorded body weights of 42 kg, at ^{224}Ra treatment and 58 kg at death, would normally have implied a marrow-free skeleton of 4.2 or 5.8 kg. However, the recorded heights of 173 cm at treatment and 176 cm at death are greater than the 170 cm height of the 70-kg reference man, whose marrow-free skeleton is 7.0 kg. (5) Scaling from reference man by height cubed (since the skeleton enlarges in all three dimensions), marrow-free skeletal weights of 7.4 or 7.8 kg seem possible. Thus, it appears likely that the marrow-free skeleton of this patient was between 7.8 and 4.2 kg, and that, consequently, his calculated average skeletal dose was between 60 and 112 rad. Therefore, it is unknown whether the dose to this sarcoma case was above or below 90 rad.

Another complication exists. It is uncertain whether this sarcoma was radiation-induced or naturally-occurring. Naturally-occurring reticulum cell sarcomas of bone are rather uncommon, constituting only 195/2962 = 6.6% of the primary malignant tumors of bone in the large series of Dahlin. (6).

In the ^{224}Ra patients of Spiess, the 55 individual bone sarcomas were diagnosed as 41 osteosarcomas, 3 chondrosarcomas, 2 polymorph cell sarcomas, 1 fibrosarcoma, 1 spindle cell sarcoma, 1 osteolytic sarcoma, *1 reticulum cell sarcoma*, and 5 unspecified sarcomas of bone. (3) Thus, while osteosarcomas have been the most frequent type of ^{224}Ra-induced bone sarcoma, other types have also occurred. In the Spiess series, the only diagnosed case of reticulum cell sarcoma occurred in Tuberculosis patient KuG, injected at age 21, in 1947-1948, with 'Peteosthor' (^{224}Ra with trace amounts of eosin and colloidal platinum). The ^{224}Ra dose is unknown, but probably high, since nearly all patients injected before 1950 received high doses. Patient KuG died 15 years after Ra treatment with a reticulum cell sarcoma of the 2nd lumbar vertebra.

Thus, it is difficult to decide whether Schales case (MaF) of reticulum cell sarcoma of bone marrow was radiation-induced or naturally-occurring, since this type of tumor has both a low natural incidence and a low induction by ^{224}Ra. However, it is important to record that it did occur.

RISK

While the bone sarcoma risk from present ^{224}Ra therapy cannot be evaluated exactly, it is possible to establish upper and lower limits. The lower limit of risk is zero, corresponding to the threshold model.

The upper limit can be derived from Poisson statistics. When the risk per individual is low (less than 10% per person) the chance P_x of having exactly 0, or 1, or 2, or ... $\underline{x}$ tumor cases when $\underline{m}$ are expected in the given population is defined by the Poisson distribution: (7)

$$P_x = \frac{m^x}{x!} e^{-m}$$

Where x factorial, or x! = 1 when x is 0 or 1,

x! = (2)(1) = 2 when x is 2

x! = (3)(2)(1) = 6 when x is 3

(a) If no bone sarcomas have occurred in the 1170 patients below 90 rad, the expected number of cases $\underline{m}$ corresponding to a 5% chance of observing none (x = 0) would be:

$$0.05 = e^{-m}$$

for which m = 3.00 expected sarcomas

(b) If 1 bone sarcoma has occurred in the 1170 patients below 90 rad, the expected number of cases m corresponding to a 5% chance of observing 1 or less (x = 1 or 0) would be:

$$0.05 = me^{-m} + e^{-m}$$

for which m = 4.74 expected sarcomas

The natural rate is about 1 bone sarcoma per year for each 100.000 persons in the German population. (8) Thus, the expected number of naturally-occurring bone sarcomas among the 1170 patients below 90 rad that have been followed an average of 12 years is:

$$[1170 \text{ persons}][12 \text{ yr}]\left[\frac{1 \text{ bone sarcoma}}{10^5 \text{ person.yr}}\right] = 0.14 \text{ natural case}$$

Therefore, the upper limit in expected ^{224}Ra-induced cases at 12 years would be 3.00 - 0.14 = 2.86 for no observed sarcomas or 4.74 - 0.14 = 4.60 for 1 observed sarcoma.

But only part of the total risk is expressed by 12 years. In the adult patients followed by Spiess, 11 bone sarcomas had appeared at 12 years, and 18 at 22 years, (3) after which the risk seems mainly exhausted. (9) Thus, the upper limits to the number of total expected cases would be (2.86)(18/11) = 4.68 cases, and (4.60)(18/11) = 7.53 cases, respectively, for zero or 1 case observed at 12 years.

The corresponding upper limits in cumulative incidence are 4.68 predicted bone sarcomas/1170 patients = 0.4%, or 7.53/1170 = 0.6%.

SUMMARY

Present evidence indicates that the bone sarcoma risk throughout lifetime, from the present ^{224}Ra therapy to adults (10 weekly injections, each of 28 μCi ^{224}Ra), is between the lower limit of 0% and the higher upper limit of 0.6%. The predicted incidence of 0.3%, from the Spiess and Mays model, (10) falls between these limits. This does not prove that the Spiess and Mays model is correct, but merely that it cannot be rejected by present data.

Only the risk from bone sarcoma has been considered in this paper. No assessment has been made of possible additional risks from ^{224}Ra, such as kidney diseases, liver diseases, and cataracts. (11)

REFERENCES

1. Schales, F., Problems and results of a new follow-up study: ^{224}Ra in adult ankylosing spondylitis patients (this symposium).
2. Spiess, H. and C.W. Mays, Bone cancers induced by ^{224}Ra (ThX) in children and adults, Health Physics 19: 713-729 (1970), plus addendum, Health Physics 20: 543-545 (1971).
3. Mays, C.W., H. Spiess and A. Gerspach, Skeletal effects following ^{224}Ra injections into humans, Health Physics (in press).
4. Schales, F., Letter to C.W. Mays (14 May 1975).
5. Snyder, W.S., M.J. Cook, L.R. Karhausen, E.S. Nasset, G.P. Howells and I.H. Tipton, *Report of the Task Group of Reference Man*, ICRP report 23, Pergamon Press, Oxford, pp. 290-291 (1975).
6. Dahlin, D.C., *Bone Tumors*, Second Edition, C.C. Thomas, publisher, Springfield, Illinois (1967).
7. Evans, R.D., *The Atomic Nucleus*, McGraw-Hill, New York, see pp. 750-753 (1955).
8. Doll, R., C. Muir and H. Waterhouse, *Cancer Incidence in Five Continents*, International Union Against Cancer, Springer-Verlag, Berlin (1970).
9. Mays, C.W. and H. Spiess, Bone sarcoma risks to man from ^{224}Ra, ^{226}Ra, and ^{239}Pu (this symposium).
10. Spiess, H. and C.W. Mays, Protraction effect on bone sarcoma induction of ^{224}Ra in children and adults, In C.L. Sanders, R.H. Busch, J.E. Ballou and

D.D. Mahlum (Ed.), *Radionuclide Carcinogenesis*, AEC Symposium Series 29, CONF-720505, pp. 437-450 (1973).
11. Spiess, H., A. Gerspach and C.W. Mays, Soft-tissue effects following ^{224}Ra injections into humans, Health Physics (in press).

Quality control in the production process and purity of ^{224}Ra for injection

Orhan Delikan, Amersham Buchler GMBH & Co. KG,
Harxbütteler Strasse 3, D 3300 Braunschweig

ABSTRACT

Buchler & Co. (since 1971 Amersham Buchler) are as far as we know the only producer of ^{224}Ra for injection. ^{224}Ra is the daughter product of ^{228}Th. We separate ^{224}Ra from ^{228}Th by a specially developed chemical method. As the long-lived radionuclides in ^{224}Ra injection are of high radiation risk to the patient, so is the quality control of these impurities in the final product of the greatest importance. The possible long-lived impurities in the ^{224}Ra solutions are ^{226}Ra, ^{228}Ra, ^{227}Ac, ^{228}Th and ^{210}Pb.

The ^{228}Th must be purified from any long-lived impurities through chemical processes before final extraction of ^{224}Ra. Only with the exact determination of the amount of these impurities the ^{228}Th can be used for the ^{224}Ra production. The amount of ^{228}Th must therefore be ascertained before release of the final product. A single injection of 28 μCi ^{224}Ra per patient weekly with a maximum total dosage of 280 μCi is recommended.

We compare the detected long-lived radioactive impurities in 280 μCi ^{224}Ra injection-solutions with the maximum values accepted by ICRP. The actual amounts of impurities present are less than 0,2% of the permissible doses recommended by ICRP.

The ^{224}Ra solution is sterilised in an autoclave to a standard corresponding to that of the national pharmacopoeia. The measurement of the ^{224}Ra solution is accomplished by evaluating the solution against a ^{226}Ra standard.

1. ^{224}RA-INJEKTIONSLÖSUNG

^{224}Ra ist das Tochternuklid des ^{228}Th und wird von ihm unter Zusatz von Calciumchlorid als Träger chemisch abgetrennt. Wir liefern das Präparat wöchentlich mit 28 μCi ^{224}Ra als Radiumchlorid (^{224}Ra) in 1 ml wässriger, sterilisierter Lösung.

Der Versand erfolgt montags mit einer maximalen Vorkalibrierung von fünf Tagen, wobei das Verfalldatum auf den sechsten Tag nach der Lieferung begrenzt wird. Diese Abgrenzung wurde wegen der Sicherstellung der Qualität bezüglich Radionuklidreinheit eingeführt, deren Grenzen von der 'International Commission on Radiological Protection' (ICRP) genau definiert sind.

2. GEFORDERTE REINHEIT DER ^{224}RA-INJEKTIONSLÖSUNG

Nach der Empfehlung der ICRP (Empfehlungen der Internationalen Kommission für Strahlenschutz, Bericht des Komitees II, 1959) liegen die maximal zulässigen Dosen bei der Inkorporation der folgenden Radionuklide bei

^{226}Ra maximal 100 nCi
^{228}Ra maximal 60 nCi
^{227}Ac maximal 30 nCi
^{228}Th maximal 20 nCi
^{210}Pb maximal 400 nCi

Um diese Grenzwerte sogar auch für Patienten einzuhalten bzw. möglichst zu unterschreiten, ist in der Herstellung und Qualitätskontrolle ein erheblicher Aufwand notwendig.

Wir überprüfen:

a. die Reinheit des einzusetzenden Mutternuklids ^{228}Th,
b. die Qualität des abgabefertigen Präparats ^{224}Ra.

Das Ausgangsprodukt ^{228}Th wird aus zusätzlichen Sicherheitsgründen erst dann zur Produktion des ^{224}Ra freigegeben, wenn die Mengen der Verunreinigungen unter 1% der von der ICRP empfohlenen Werte liegen.

3. DIE QUALITäTSKONTROLLE

Wir überprüfen die Qualität der ^{224}Ra-Lösung nach folgenden Methoden:

3.1. Die Kontrolle der Reinheit des Mutternuklids ^{228}Th

Die Reinheit der ^{224}Ra-Injektionslösung ist von der Qualität des Ausgangsstoffes ^{228}Th abhängig. Das ^{228}Th kann je nach seiner Herstellungsmethode die Radionuklide ^{226}Ra, ^{228}Ra, ^{227}Ac, ^{210}Pb enthalten. Diese Radionuklide bzw. ihre Tochternuklide dürfen bei der Herstellung des ^{224}Ra nicht in die Injektionslösung gelangen. Das ^{228}Th wird deshalb vor seinem Einsatz von diesen Verunreinigungen durch chemische Prozesse gereinigt. Zur Herstellung der Analysenprobe wird das ^{228}Th mit ^{232}Th geträgert und als Thoriumhydroxid ausgefällt. Daraus wird das ^{224}Ra durch Extraktion unter Zusatz von Calciumchlorid als Trägermaterial abgetrennt.

Für die Analyse werden mehrere Proben zu je 1 mCi ^{224}Ra in Ampullen eingeschlossen. Nach drei Monaten ist die ^{224}Ra-Aktivität abgeklungen. Erst nach Ablauf dieser Zeit ist die quantitative Erfassung der langlebigen Verunreinigungen möglich.

Die Bestimmung der Fremdnuklide erfolgt durch γ-spektrometrische Messungen

a. bei uns
b. zusätzlich bei der Physikalisch-Technischen-Bundesanstalt in Braunschweig.

Sind die Mengen der Verunreinigungen unter 1% der ICRP-Werte so wird das ^{228}Th zur Produktion freigegeben. Liegen die Werte darüber, so erfolgt ein nochmaliger Reinigungsprozess des ^{228}Th.

3.2 Die Überprüfung des ^{228}Th-Gehaltes in der abgabefertigen ^{224}Ra-Injektionslösung

Um sicherzustellen, dass in der ^{224}Ra-Injektionslösung weniger als die zulässige Menge ^{228}Th enthalten ist, werden von jeder Produktionscharge Proben mit je 1 mCi ^{224}Ra nach einer von uns entwickelten Methode auf Reinheit bezüglich des ^{228}Th-Gehaltes geprüft. Zu diesem Zweck werden die Proben mit Lösungen von Thorium-, Blei-, Barium- und Wismutnitrat geträgert. Durch Zusatz von 2 N Schwefelsäure werden die Folgeprodukte der in der Zerfallsreihe unter dem ^{228}Th stehenden Elemente als Sulfate ausgefällt (Abbildung Thorium Zerfallsreihe). Nach wiederholten Fällungen verbleibt das zu bestimmende, geträgerte ^{228}Th in der Lösung. Durch die Messung des nachwachsenden Folgeproduktes ^{212}Pb über seine bei 0,239 MeV liegende γ-Energie wird der Gehalt an ^{228}Th bestimmt. Die Nachweisgrenze dieser Analysenmethode beträgt 1% des maximal zulässigen Wertes von 20 nCi für das ^{228}Th.

3.3. Die Messung der ^{224}Ra-Aktivität

Die Aktivitätsmessung des ^{224}Ra erfolgt in einer kalibrierten Ionisationskammer. Es wird die Gammastrahlung der Folgeprodukte des ^{224}Ra gemessen. Zur Geräteüberprüfung und Eichung wird ein ^{226}Ra-Standard verwendet.

3.4. Die Prüfung auf Sterilität und Pyrogenfreiheit

Die ^{224}Ra-Lösung wird vor der Abfüllung durch einen Filter mit 5 μm Porengrösse gereinigt. Die abgefüllten Flaschen werden bei einem Druck von 1,1 atü und einer Temperatur von 120°C dampfsterilisiert.

Die Prüfung auf die Sterilität der Lösung erfolgt nach dem Deutschen Arzneibuch DAB 7.

4. ERGEBNISSE

Die Mengen der einzelnen Verunreinigungen in der ^{224}Ra-Lösung werden auf 280 μCi ^{224}Ra bezogen, weil dem Verwender empfohlen wird, pro Patient maximal 10 Einzeldosen mit insgesamt 280 μCi ^{224}Ra, verteilt über 10 Wochen zu injizieren. Durch die Überprüfung der Verunreinigungen im Mutter-

Thorium - Zerfallsreihe

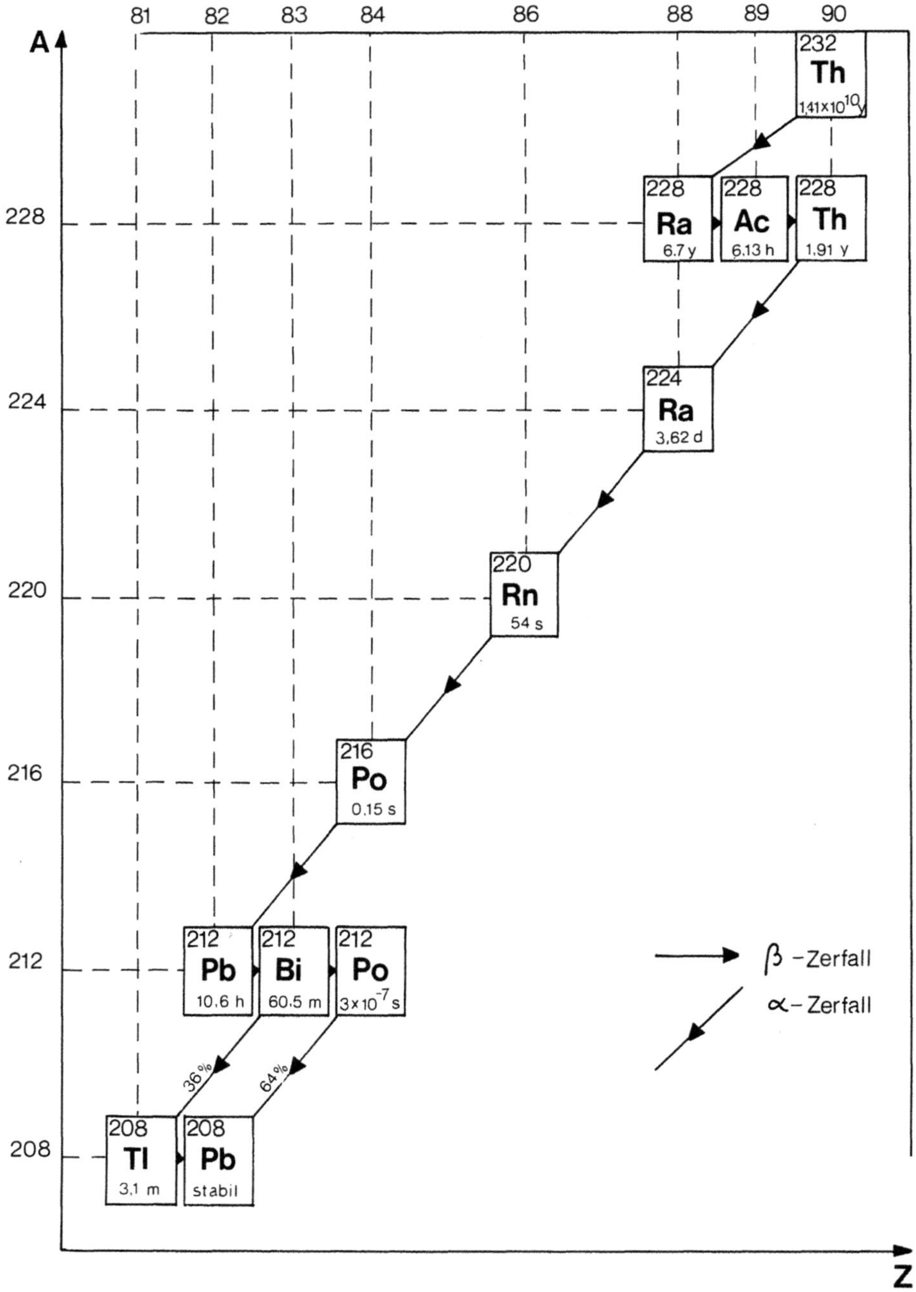

nuklid ^{228}Th wird erreicht, dass nur hochreines ^{228}Th zum Einsatz kommt.

In der folgenden Tabelle sind die quantitativ erfassten maximalen Mengen an langlebigen Verunreinigungen in der ^{224}Ra-Lösung wiedergegeben. Der Vergleich mit den maximal zulässigen Mengen der Fremdnuklide nach ICRP, bezogen auf die entsprechenden kritischen Organe zeigt, dass der Patient nach der Behandlung mit 280 µCi ^{224}Ra einer maximalen Strahlenbelastung von nur 0,03% für ^{226}Ra bis 0,17% für ^{228}Th der von der ICRP als zulässig erkannten Werte ausgesetzt wird.

TABEL

Radio-nuklid	Kritisches Organ	Max.zulässige Belastung nach ICRP	In 280 µCi ^{224}Ra sind maximal enthalten	Die erfasste Menge in % der max. zulässigen Belastung
^{226}Ra	Knochen	100 nCi	0,034 nCi	0,03 %
^{228}Ra	Knochen	60 nCi	0,018 nCi	0,03 %
^{227}Ac	Knochen	30 nCi	0,035 nCi	0,12 %
^{210}Pb	Niere	400 nCi	0,034 nCi	0,01 %
^{228}Th	Knochen	20 nCi	0,034 nCi	0,17 %

Durch den erheblichen Aufwand in der Qualitätskontrolle bei uns wird sichergestellt, dass durch die Injektion des ^{224}Ra-Präparates keine zusätzliche, unzulässige Strahlenbelastung des Patienten auftritt.

Es kann heute gesagt werden, dass vom Standpunkt der Strahlenbelastung durch die unerwünschten langlebigen Nuklide gegen den Einsatz von ^{224}Ra als Radiotherapeutikum beim derzeitigen Stande unseres Wissens keine Einwände zu bestehen brauchen.

Therapeutical results in a follow-up study on ^{224}Ra-therapy of ankylosing spondylitis

E. Schmitt, Orthopädische Universitätsklinik Friedrichsheim Frankfurt/Main-Niederrad, Marienburgstrasse 2, Federal Republic of Germany

ABSTRACT

From 1952 to 1970 in the Universitätsklinik Friedrichsheim, Frankfurt am Main, about 200 patients were treated with Thorium-X because of Morbus Bechterew. It was possible to re-examine 80 in 200 patients clinically, by röntgenology and in laboratory; additionally 49 of them were explored by questionnaire. In 70 per cent of the cases a lasting subjective recovery occurred and the inflammatory activities were reduced. You can see clearly these results in comparison to a collective of patients, which was attended without Thorium-X. After treatment during the same period one could ascertain in this group a higher inflammatory activity. The subjective complaints decreased continuously only for 19%. In comparison to this, the clinical and röntgenological statement showed no differences. There were no references to damage by radioactivity in any of the cases.

In Zusammenarbeit mit der Gesellschaft für Strahlen- und Umweltforschung und den Orthopädischen Universitätskliniken Münster, Hannover, Kiel, Köln, Würzburg und Frankfurt/Main wurde eine Studie über den Effekt der Thorium-X-Behandlung beim Morbus Bechterew durchgeführt. Teilergebnisse aus der Frankfurter Klinik liegen jetzt vor.

Bis 1946 war die Therapie des Bechterew in Deutschland rein symptomatisch. In grundlegenden Arbeiten von Troch, Pitzen und vor allem Koch gibt es jetzt eine gezielte Strahlentherapie: Thorium-X und seine Folgeprodukte, so zeigte Koch, wirken antiosteoplastisch und stören alle in Ausbildung begriffenen enchondralen und endesmalen Verknöcherungsprozesse. Seitdem ist auch eine Vielzahl von Arbeiten zu diesem Thema erschienen, von denen nur einige neue zitiert werden sollen:

Laschner berichtete 1973 über 81 von 109 zwischen 1976 und 1971 mit Thorium-X behandelten Patienten. Subjektive Schmerzlinderung, objektive Zunahme der Beweglichkeit sind positive Effekte. Er findet aber auch bei einer grossen Zahl Störungen der Serum-Labilitätsproben.

Laschner und Schüler fanden 1969 bei 133 Patienten sehr gute Ergebnisse mit jahrelanger Schmerzlinderung und Zunahme der Beweglichkeit. Die Hälfte dieses Kollektivs bezeichnet das Thorium-X als wirksamste Therapie überhaupt.

Wichtig sind ferner Arbeiten von Koch und Kutz, Hertel und Heine, 1974.

Daneben gibt es aber auch Veröffentlichungen, die sich sehr kritisch zur Thorium-X-Wirkung und vor allem deren Nebeneffekten äussern. Stieglitz u.a. berichten 1973 über eine Schädigung der Hämatopoese durch Thorium-X. Sie geben die Epikrise von zwei Patienten wieder, die bei Dosen von 2400 elektrostatischen Einheiten, verteilt über 12 Wochen, 7 bzw. 11 Jahre nach der Behandlung eine Paraplastenleukose bzw. Myelopathie bekamen und verstarben. Die Autoren vergleichen diese Krankengeschichten mit anderen und bringen eine Zusammenfassung der Literatur: Von 1952 bis 1968 verstarben 13 Patienten an einer hämatologischen Erkrankung nach Thorium-X. Die Gesamtdosen pro Patient schwanken aber erheblich (200 bis ingesamt 22000 elektrostatische Einheiten). Ein sicherer Zusammenhang zwischen Dosis und Erkrankung ist also nich sicher zu erkennen.

Thiele und Stieglitz machen deshalb den Vorschlag, regelmässig hämatologische Kontrolluntersuchungen durchzuführen (Hb, Retikulocytenzahl, Leukocytenzahl, Differential-Blutbild,

Stauversuch nach Rümpfel-Lede) 1973.

Knoop (1974) fand ein Schilddrüsen-Carcinom nach X-Thor, allerdings bei einem Kind. Honeger berichtet über einen doppelseitigen Strahlenkatarakt nach Peteostor.

Schliesslich soll noch einmal Kutz zitiert werden, der schon 1956 über Kernatypien im Sternalpunktat berichtete, die aber vorwiegend dann auftraten, wenn wöchentlich zweimal 200 elektrostatische Einheiten gegeben wurden. Nach Reduzierung der Dosis auf eine Injektion pro Woche sinkt die Anzahl der Patienten, die Kernatypien aufweisen. Es gibt zu diesem Thema frühere Äusserungen von Koch und Schales: Bei diesen Atypien handele es sich um flüchtige Erscheinungen, sie stellen keine bleibende Veränderung dar.

Bei Durchsicht der klinischen Arbeiten werden immer wieder zwei kardinale Fragen gestellt:

1. Wie gross ist das wahre Ausmass des positiven Effektes des Thorium-X beim Morbus Bechterew in subjektiver und objektiver Hinsicht? Überwiegen die Vorteile dieser Behandlung gegenüber einer medikamentösen oder einer anderen Strahlenbehandlung?
2. Welches Risiko geht man mit dieser Behandlung ein? Dabei sollten aber nicht Massstäbe des allgemeinen Risikos der Strahlenbehandlung angelegt werden, sondern man muss die besondere Situation des Bechterew-Kranken mit seinem schweren Schicksal berücksichtigen.

1952 wurde das Thorium-X in der Frankfurter Klinik eingeführt. Seit dieser Zeit bis 1970 konnten 200 Patienten mit Thorium-X behandelt werden. Kutz berichtete 1965 und 1963 bereits über Ergebnisse an 92 dieser Patienten. Seit 1957 ist es üblich einmal pro Woche eine Injektion mit 200 elektrostatischen Einheiten Thorium-X zu verabfolgen, das entspricht nach der Umrechnung von Schales 25 bis 28 mikrocurie pro Woche. Zusätzlich werden physikalische Massnahmen, nach Bedarf auch Analgetica verordnet.

Im fraglichen Zeitraum verstarben 26 Patienten des Kollektivs. Wir haben Mitteilungen nur von Gesundheitsämtern auswerten können, leider liegen keine Sektionsbefunde vor. Deshalb sind die Angaben teilweise ungenau. 12 Patienten starben an einem Herz-Kreislaufversagen, 6 davon an einem Infarkt, 3 an einer Erkrankung der Lunge, je 1 an einer Nierenerkrankung und Arteriosklerose, 2 an Kachexie, 2 durch Unfall, 1 Patient durch Suizid, 3 an einem Malignom aber ohne nähere Bezeichnung, 1 Patient verstarb an einer Panmyelopathie, dieser wurde aber vor 1952 ausserdem mit Peteostor behandelt.

129 Patienten des Kollektivs wurden anhand eines ausführlichen Fragebogens exploriert. Hier soll nur auf die Fragen eingegangen werden, die in diesem Zusammenhang von Relevanz sind:

TABELLE I

Kein X-Thor N= 80		X-Thor N= 129
37 - 46,2 %	Keine Besserung	34 - 26,3 %
38 - 47,5 %	Vorübergehende Besserung	28 - 21,7 %
5 - 6,3 %	Länger anhaltende Besserung	67 - 52,0 %

Bei der Auswertung des Fragebögen konnte bei 80 Patienten ein direkter Vergleich des Thorium-X-Effektes mit anderen Behandlungsmöglichkeiten gezogen werden (ausschliesslich physikalische Therapie, Röntgenbestrahlung, Medikamente, keine Behandlung), vergl. Tabel I. Kein Erfolg der Nicht-Thorium-X-Behandelten trat bei 46,2%, eine vorübergehende Besserung bei 47,5, eine längere Besserung nur bei 6,3% ein. Bei 19 von 80 Patienten musste ein Tablettenmissbrauch angenommen werden. Alle diese Patienten erhielten später Thorium-X und bezeichneten diese Behandlung als wesentlich wirksamer. Unter insgesamt 129 derartig behandelter Patienten trat eine langanhaltende Besserung bei 52%, eine vorübergehende Besserung bei 21,7%, keine Besserung bei 17,8% auf.

Die Patienten differenzierten auch die Qualität der Besserung: Die Hälfte gab eine Schmerzlinderung, die andere Hälfte eine Zunahme der Beweglichkeit an.

18 Unter diesen 129 Patienten zeugten noch Kinder nach der Thorium-X-Behandelung, es waren ingesammt 27 (11 x 1, 2 x 2, 1 x 3, 1 x 4). 22 Kinder waren zum Zeitpunkt der

Untersuchung völlig gesund, 5 krank, hatten aber keine Veränderungen, die als Strahlenschaden zu bezeichnen sind.

80 Patienten konnten ausserdem klinisch und röntgenologisch nachuntersucht werden. Wir hatten die Gelegenheit, auch Blutproben zu entnehmen. Diese Nachuntersuchungen fanden zwischen einem und 20 Jahren nach der Thorium-X-Behandlung statt: Im Mittel 10,3 Jahre.

0 - 5 Jahre	14	Patienten
6 - 10 Jahre	22	Patienten
11 - 15 Jahre	32	Patienten
16 - 20 Jahre	11	Patienten
21 - 25 Jahre	1	Patient.

7 Von diesen Patienten erhielten 2 X-Thor-Kuren, 3 bekamen vor dieser Behandlung Peteostor. Einmal musste die Behandlung wegen Unverträglichkeit (ohne nähere Angaben) abgebrochen werden.

Sehr informativ sind die Äusserungen zum Effekt. Es liegen 78 verwertbare Aussagen vor: Unmittelbar nach der Behandlung gaben 79,5% eine Besserung an, zwei Jahre danach betrug die Besserungsrate noch 75,6%, verschlechtert hatten sich 1,3%. Bei der Nachuntersuchung (im Schnitt 10,2 Jahre) fühlten sich noch besser 70,5%, schlechter dagegen 5,1%. Dauer des X-Thor-Effektes N= 78:

TABELLE II

	Unmittelbar N %	2 Jahre nach X-Thor N %	Nach-Untersuchung N %
Besser	62 - 79,5	59 - 75,6	55 - 70,5
Gleich		18 - 23,1	19 - 24,4
Schlechter		1 - 1,3	4 - 5,1

Anders sieht es bei den klinischen Werten aus (N= 76). 4 Parameter wurden herausgesucht, die für den Bechterew typisch sind: Die Halswirbelsäulenbeweglichkeit war unter diesen 76 Patienten nur 11 mal ungestört, 18 hatten eine komplete Versteifung der Halswirbelsäule. Das Schober'sche Zeichen und die Atembreite waren bei allen Patienten eingeschränkt. Eine Beteiligung der Hüftgelenke war in 63

Fällen feststellbar, nur 14 hatten eine freie Hüftgelenksbeweglichkeit.

Signifikante Werte konnten auch bei den Laboruntersuchungen nicht festgestellt werden. Das Gesamteiweiss lag bei 57 von 76 Patienten im Normbereich, 9 mal war es leicht vermindert (zwischen 5,95 und 6,44 und einmal mit 8,9 erhöht, dies stellt keine signifikante Abweichung dar). Bei der Elektrophorese war in 1/3 der Fälle eine Gamma-Globulin-Erhöhung feststellbar, entsprechend einer chronischen Entzündung. Blutbild, Hämoglobin, Erythrocytenzahl, Form und Zahl der Leukocyten zeigten keine verwertbaren Veränderungen. Die alkalische Phosphatase lag bei 63 von 71 Patienten im Normbereich, deutlich erhöht nur bei 8. SGOT und SGPT waren 65 mal (von 70) normal. Diese Ergebnisse zeigen, dass eine typische Störung nicht vorliegt.

Deutlichere Hinweise ergeben sich durch die Blutsenkungsgeschwindigkeit: Bei 65 Patienten befand sich 22 mal die BSG im Normbereich, bei 43 erhöht (Verhältnis etwa 1 : 2).

Das bedeutet, dass nach den Standarduntersuchungsmethoden keine konkreten Hinweise für eine Störung der Hämatopoese oder der Leber festgestellt wurden. Trotz erhöhter entzündlicher Aktivitäten (bei 2/3 der Patienten) ist das subjektive Befinden besser (3/4 der Patienten).

Bei der Beurteilung der Röntgenaufnahmen ging man davon aus, ob seit der Thorium-X-Behandlung radiologisch der Bechterew stehen geblieben war oder ob er sich wenig oder stark verschlechterte. Eine Progredienz war nicht mehr nachweisbar bei 7 von 70 Patienten, eine mässige Verschlechterung bei 14, eine deutliche Verschlechterung bis hin zum Endstadium bei 49 Patienten.

Offensichtlich besteht also eine Diskrepanz zwischen den subjektiven Angaben und den objektiven klinischen und röntgenologischen Befunden. Trotz Erleichterung und Zufriedenheit schreitet der Bechterew in einem hohen Prozentsatz weiter fort.

Zusätzlich konnten auch 70 Patienten nachuntersucht werden, die im gleichen Zeitraum wegen eines Morbus Bechterew stationär aber ohne Thorium-X behandelt worden waren (1952 bis

1970). Soweit vertretbar und zulässig, sind auch direkte Vergleiche angestellt worden. Diesbezüglich wird die Sammelstatistik aller Kliniken grössere Relevanz besitzen. Trotz eingeschränkter Aussagewerte lassen sich aber deutlich Tendenzen erkennen, so z.B. in den Äusserungen der Patienten bzgl. ihres Befindens zur Zeit der Befragung. Besser nach der Behandlung fühlten sich 14 von 70 (19,9%), gleichbleibend 51 (72,9%), schlechter 5 (7,2%). Das Verhältnis 'besser' zu 'gleichbleibend' ist also im Vergleich zu den Thorium-X-Behandelten umgekehrt:

TABELLE III

NACHUNTERSUCHUNGEN

(DURCHSCHNITTLICH 10,2 JAHRE NACH BEHANDLUNG)

Kein X-Thor N= 80		X-Thor N= 129
14 - 19,9 %	Besser	55 - 70,5 %
51 - 72,9 %	Gleichbleibend	19 - 24,4 %
5 - 7,2 %	Schlechter	4 - 15,1 %

Kein Unterschied ergibt sich dagegen bei den klinischen Befunden. Die Halswirbelsäulenfunktion war in diesem Kollektiv nur einmal frei (16 mal totale Versteifung). Das Schober'sche Zeichen war bei allen pathologisch, die Atembreite nur bei 3 normal. Die Hüftgelenke waren in 54 Fällen mitbeteiligt, nur 16 mal ohne klinisch nachweisbare Einschränkung:

TABELLE IV

BEWEGLICHKEITSEINSCHRÄNKUNG

Kein X-Thor N= 70		X-Thor N= 76
69 - 98,6 %	Halswirbelsäule	65 - 85,5 %
70 - 100 %	Schober	76 - 100 %
67 - 96,7 %	Atembreite	76 - 100 %
54 - 77,1 %	Hüftfunktion	62 - 81,6 %

Die Untersuchung der Blutwerte erbrachte unter 49 Patienten 46 mal eine normale alkalische Phosphatase, nur 3 mal eine Erhöhung, die BSG war bei 48 Patienten 10 mal normal und 38 mal erhöht (Verhältnis 1 : 4). Auch die übrigen Laborwerte zeigen keine verwertbare Veränderung:

TABELLE V

Kein X-Thor N= 48 normal	erhöht	X-Thor N= 65 normal	erhöht
10	38	22	43
0,263		0,512	

Die Auswertung der Röntgenbilder ergibt ebenfalls keinen Hinweis auf differentes Verhalten:

TABELLE VI

Kein X-Thor N= 54		X-Thor N= 70
7	Stehengeblieben	7
6	Wenig weiterentwickelt	14
41	Deutlich weiterentwickelt	49
1 : 6,7	Verhältnis Stillstand : Weiterentwicklung	1 : 9

Von 54 Patienten ist 7 mal der Röntgenbefund nicht schlechter geworden, 6 mal wenig schlechter und 41 mal stark verschlechtert.

Zusammenfassend ist also festzustellen, dass nach Thorium-es 70% der Patienten subjektiv besser geht, nur 5% schlechter. Man stellt auch einen Rückgang der entzündlichen Aktivitäten, durch die BSG ausgedrückt, fest. Patienten, die nicht mit Thorium-X behandelt worden sind, konnten nur zu 19,9% gebessert werden, 7% ging es schlechter. Der Anteil der Patienten, die eine erhöhte BSG hatten, ist in dieser Vergleichsgruppe höher. Dagegen enttäuscht der Vergleich 'klinische und röntgenologische Befunde'. Wesentliche Unterschiede zwischen diesen beiden Patientengruppen bestehen hier nicht. Wichtig ist aber, dass mit den üblichen Methoden der Klinik und des Labors und der Röntgenologie Strahlenschäden nicht festgestellt werden konnten.

Damit wird der Wert des Thorium-X als Therapeuticum beim Morbus Bechterew bestätigt. Die Schmerzhaftigkeit nimmt deutlicher und länger anhaltend ab als im Vergleich zu anderen Medikamenten. Es vollzieht sich ein protrahierter und gemilderter Verlauf. Nimmt man die Erfahrungen anderer Untersucher hinzu, so muss auch festgestellt werden, dass die Beweglichkeit unmittelbar nach der Thorium-X-Behandlung besser ist als mit Vergleichsbehandlungen. Die Gefahr des Strahlenschadens ist nach dieser Untersuchung äusserst gering. Berücksichtigt man zusätzlich, dass alle anderen beim Bechterew gebräuchlichen Medikamente unerwünschte Nebenwirkungen besitzen und zum Teil schwere, irreparabele Schädigungen hervorrufen, dann ergibt sich durch den Gebrauch des Thorium-X kein erhöhtes Risiko. Freilich ist bei der Therapie mit diesem Alpha-Strahler, das beweist die Geschichte des Thorium-X selbst, eine strenge Indikation und eine exakte Dosierung einzuhalten.

LITERATURVERZEICHNIS

1. Barth, G., S.F. Grebe und F. Schales, Zur Kritik der Strahlenbehandlung bei ankylosierender Spondylitis, Verh.Dtsch.Ges.Rheumatol. 1, 149-55 (1969).
2. Becker, F., C. Lepp, H. Peomsl und A. Luz, Störung des Knochenwachstums nach Inkorporation von RA-224 (Thorium-X) bei der Maus, Verh.Dtsch.Ges.Pathol.56, 448-52 (1972).
3. Gössner, W., Grundlagen und allgemeine pathologische Anatomie der Strahlenschäden, Verh.Dtsch.Ges.Pathol. 56, 168-87 (1972).
4. Gössner, W., B. Hindringer, O. Hug, A. Luz und W.A. Müller, Spätschäden nach Inkorporation von RA-224 im Tierexperiment, Fortschr.Geb.Röntgenstr.Nuklearmed.Suppl.149-50 (1972)

5. Hertel, E. und J. Heine, Sakroiliakaler Strontium-Umsatz und Thorium-X-Therapie bei Morbus Bechterew, Z.Orthop. 112, 842-5, (Aug. 1974).
6. Honeger, H., Strahlenkatarakt nach Peteosthorbehandlung (Thorium-X), Klin.Monatsbl.Augenheilkd. 155, 890-5, (Dez. 1969).
7. Knoop, U. und D. Genz, Lungenmetastasen durch Schilddrüsencarcinom im Kindesalter nach Thorium-X-Behandlung, Z.Kinderheilkd. 118, 117-27 (1974).
8. Koch, W., Ergebnisse einer zwanzigjährigen parenteralen Thorium-X-Therapie der knöchern-entzündlichen Wirbelsäulenversteifung (Morbus Bechterew), Verh.Dtsch.Ges. Rheumatol. 1, 132-40 (1969).
9. Laschner, W., Ergebnisse und Komplikationen der Thorium-X-Behandlung bei Morbus Bechterew, Z.Orthop. 111, 743-8, (Okt. 1973).
10. Laschner, W. und W. Arnold, Zur Therapie der Spondylitis ankylopoetica (Indikation zur Thorium-X-Therapie), Beitr.Orthop.Traumatol. 18, 24-6 (1971).
11. Luz, A. und B. Hindringer, Ossifizierende Kifer-Fibrome bei der Maus nach Inkorporation von RA-224 (Thorium-X), Verh.Dtsch.Ges.Pathol. 54, 450-4 (1970).
12. Schales, F., Zur Strahlentherapie der Spondylarthritis ankylopoetica, Z.Orthop. 106, 798-805, (Sept. 1969).
13. Schales, F. und D.E. Jones, The Specification of Thorium-X Activity: The E.S.U. to Curie Conversion, Br.J.Radiol. 43, 471-8, (Juli 1970).
14. Stieglitz, R., M. Thiele, H. Stobbe und G. Wegener, Schädigungen der Hämatopoese durch Thorium-X-Therapie, Folia Haematol. (Leipz.) 100, 95-103 (1973).
15. Thiele, M., R. Stieglitz, H. Stobbe und G. Wegener, Vorschlag eines Programms hämatologischer Kontrolluntersuchungen bei der Thorium-X-Therapie des Morbus Bechterew, Beitr.Orthop.Traumatol. 20, 310-5, (Juni 1973).

X-Ray therapy in the treatment of ankylosing spondylitis

Sir Brian Windeyer, National Radiological Protection Board, Harwell, Didcot, Oxon OX11 ORQ, England

ABSTRACT

This contribution is based on the treatment by X-rays of 1432 patients diagnosed as suffering from ankylosing spondylitis during the years 1939 to 1955 at the Middlesex Hospital London.

From among them a randomly selected series of 277 patients was chosen and details are presented of the age and sex distribution and the clinical stage of the disease. The variations in presenting features and the diagnostic criteria are discussed in relation to the details of the techniques of X-ray therapy and ancillary treatment employed.

The results of the treatment of this series of patients is presented and some consideration is given to the complications and sequelae of the X-ray therapy here described. There is particular reference to the risk of leukaemogenesis, the decline in the use of X-ray therapy and the present position in Britain of the management of ankylosing spondylitis.

X-RAY THERAPY IN THE TREATMENT OF ANKYLOSING SPONDYLITIS

I have to make some explanation of why I, who retired from the active practice of radiotherapy seven years ago, have come to speak to this Symposium about a series of patients who were treated more than twenty years ago. It is because

I did have the opportunity of treating by X-rays a relatively large number of patients suffering from ankylosing spondylitis and because this method of treatment became unpopular in Britain following the discovery of the leukaemogenic effects of radiotherapy so that radiotherapists at the present time treat only occasional patients.

Between the years 1939 and 1955 some 1430 patients suffering from ankylosing spondylitis were treated by X-ray therapy at the Middlesex Hospital and Mount Vernon Hospital where I was in charge. This period included the war years and as at that time it was considered that X-ray therapy was the method of choice for the treatment of this disease, the majority of Service personnel were referred to a relatively limited number of centres and I received a high proportion of those from London and nearby. This number does in fact represent about one-tenth of those in the series of Court Brown and Doll, whose investigation was started by the Medical Research Council during the preparation of the report on the Hazards to Man of Nuclear and Allied Radiations. It began from a report by van Swaay of Leiden of the development of leukaemia and aplastic anaemia in seven patients who had been treated by X-rays for ankylosing spondylitis and of the development of leukaemia in two of my first 1000 patients.

It was not possible, mainly due to the difficulties of the times, to make a complete follow-up of all patients treated but I did examine the records of a series of 277 patients, chosen at random, and which appeared to be fairly representative of the whole; there were 255 males and 22 females. That is, 92 per cent were male and 8 per cent female.

The age incidence was as follows:

Under 20 years	6 =	2.2 %
20 - 29	100 =	37.0 %
30 - 39	115 =	42.5 %
40 - 49	36 =	13.2 %
50 - 59	10 =	3.7 %
60 - 70	4 =	1.4 %

The patients were divided into three clinical stages according to the degree of involvement of the spine, and for this assessment account was taken of the symptoms of pain and a subjective feeling of stiffness as well as the sign of restriction of movement.

Stage I	Active disease localised to the sacro-iliac and lumbar regions
Stage II	Active disease affecting the whole or most of the spine but with little or no calcification of ligaments
Stage III	Active disease which has affected the whole or most of the spine and there is extensive calcification of ligaments.

The assessment was made before any treatment was commenced.

Stage I	48 patients	17.3 %
Stage II	181 patients	65.4 %
Stage III	48 patients	17.3 %

This classification was adopted in an attempt to determine the results of treatment with some correlation with the severity of the disease. It was realised that it is a relatively crude method of classification as there are many patients in whom the disease is not at all typical in its distribution. There are some in whom pain, stiffness and even ligamentous calcification commence in the cervical or in the thoracic part of the spine without obvious disease in the lumbar spine or sacro-iliac joints. There are others in whom the disease commences as an acute fever, perhaps with pain in various muscle groups such as the latissimus dorsi or the pectorals, and there are others who have involvement of peripheral joints before there are any symptoms or signs referable to the spine or sacro-iliac region.

The incidence of involvement of peripheral joints and of muscle attachments to bone was assessed in each of these stages, the evidence of involvement being radiological changes and symptoms of such severity that X-ray therapy was given.

Stage I	48 patients	13 or 27 % with bones and/or joints
Stage II	181 patients	55 or 31 % with bones and/or joints
Stage III	48 patients	32 or 68 % with bones and/or joints

It can be seen that in the 277 cases there was peripheral joint or bone involvement in 100 and that even in Stage I, more than one-quarter of the patients had such involvement outside the spine. With more advanced spinal disease the incidence of peripheral bone and joint involvement becomes much greater. In the 277 cases the following bones and joints were affected:

Hips	60 times	Ischial tuberosity	22 times
Knees	26 times	Iliac crest	9 times
Shoulder	22 times	Symphysis pubis	4 times
Temporo-mandibular	1 time	Great Trochanter	3 times
Sterno-clavicular	1 time	Scapula	1 time
Acromio-clavicular	1 time	Os calcis	7 times
Wrist	3 times	Costal cartilages	1 time
Ankle	1 time	Femoral condyle	1 time

DIAGNOSIS

Although the problems of diagnosis and natural history of this disease have already been dealt with this morning, I think that I must say something about my concepts of these topics in explanation of the basis of the X-ray therapy that we have used.

The diagnosis of ankylosing spondylitis in patients with advanced disease is obviously reasonably simple and straightforward, but in the earlier stages there may be great difficulty. The symptoms and signs may simulate other diseases to such an extent that the diagnosis may be missed for months or even years. On the other hand, at a time when it was considered that X-ray therapy was a useful method of treatment and that the best results were obtained when there was early recognition and early treatment, there were a number of patients who were referred for radiotherapy with a diagnosis of early ankylosing spondylitis who did not have this disease but were suffering from some other undiagnosed condition.

The diagnosis used to rest on the clinical findings and on the radiological appearances and close correlation of them both was necessary. Since my time there has been the additional factor of the recognition of the specific genetic antigen present in patients suffering from ankylosing spondylitis and Reiter's Syndrome.

In the typical early case the history of pain and stiffness in the lower back, perhaps intermittent in character, associated with muscle spasm of the long lumbar muscles and the radiological appearance of osteoporosis, erosion and absorption of the sacro-iliac joint margins with perhaps a band of sclerosis outside them, made the diagnosis quite certain.

But there are many variations of this theme. Rarely the pain, stiffness and spasm may originate in the neck or the thorax with diminution of chest expansion and with minimal signs in the lumbar region.

In some patients the disease may present as an acute infectious process. There may be pyrexia of unknown origin, marked asthenia, loss of appetite, night sweats, and generalised pains in joints and muscles.

I believe that there are some patients who, following trauma, develop pain in the sacro-iliac joint and have radiological appearances, predominantly of sclerosis around the joint margins, which may be confused with ankylosing spondylitis.

In the elderly there is a tendency to ankylosis of the sacro-iliac joints and this, combined with the heavy sharp spurs of osteoarthritis of the spine, may also give rise to mistakes in diagnosis.

In going through our records we found that those patients in whom there was some doubt about the diagnosis invariably had the least successful result from treatment. It was a matter of some importance that radiotherapy, which is not a simple treatment and which may have dangerous sequelae should be reserved for the treatment of those conditions which it will really benefit.

The erythrocyte sedimentation rate is variable in ankylosing spondylitis. We have seen readings as high as 80 in the first hour in patients who did not have severe symptoms and whose disease appeared on clinical examination to be almost inactive. There have been others with quite acute disease in whom the sedimentation rate has been raised hardly above normal. We found difficulty in correlating the sedimentation rate readings with the results of treatment.

TREATMENT

In Britain, X-ray therapy had an important part to play in the treatment of ankylosing spondylitis. In fact it is probably true to say that this form of treatment revolutionised the immediate general outlook and the long-term prognosis of the patient with this disease. Radiotherapy is, however, only one part of the proper treatment, which may have to include efficient orthopaedic treatment, general medical treatment and well-conducted and sometimes prolonged physiotherapy. General supportive treatment is necessary to improve appetite and nutrition, to promote rest and sleep and sometimes to correct anaemia.

The type of orthopaedic treatment which is desirable used to give rise to considerable discussion. Before radiotherapy was used to any extent in ankylosing spondylitis it was customary to immobilise patients with plaster collars, plaster jackets and plaster beds, on the basis that when the inevitable ankylosis had occurred it would be in the best possible position and with the least possible contracture and deformity. It was also necessary in many cases to immobilise in this way in order to reduce spasm and relieve pain. The outstanding immediate effect of X-ray therapy is the reduction of muscle spasm and the relief of pain.

It is then possible to begin movements and to restore function.

When X-ray therapy is used it is not necessary and it is inadvisable to carry out prolonged immobilisation, but it may be necessary to have some plaster or other orthopaedic appliance at the beginning of treatment to promote rest, reduce spasm and prevent further deformity from the stretching of inefficient muscles until the X-ray treatment has begun to be effective and until various muscle groups have been re-educated and restored. Fracture boards should be used to keep the bed straight and a plaster bed may be necessary to allow adequate rest during the course of treatment.

X-ray therapy was indicated in all cases where there were any symptoms of activity of the disease. Some patients have spontaneous remission at any stage, and this may apparently be permanent. There is no object in giving X-ray treatment when there is no activity. But there are some patients with advanced disease and complete ankylosing of the spine, with the bamboo radiological appearance in Stage III of my classification who may still have activity with pain and muscle spasm. Radiotherapy will then relieve discomfort; even in these advanced cases it will procure some improvement in movement through reduction of spasm and may prevent further immobilisation, perhaps of the atlanto-occipital joint, the only one which remains free.

The technique which we evolved was to use X-rays generated at 200-250 kilovolts with a quality of radiation expressed in terms of 2 mm. Cu. half value layer. The usual fields with 40 cm. anode skin distance were:

1. Sacro-iliac joints	10 x 15 sq. cms
2. Lumbar spine	7.5 x 15 sq. cms
3. Dorsal spine	7.5 x 15 sq. cms
4. Dorso-cervical spine	7.5 x 15 sq. cms

The dose given to each field was 2000 roentgens, measured on the skin, delivered over a period of four weeks. This produced a mild erythema with some subsequent pigmentation.

In Britain, X-ray therapy for this and other diseases affecting joints used to be given by small doses of, say, 100 rads repeated at intervals of one or more weeks, but the new generation of radiotherapists appearing in the early 1930s considered that a single fractionated course of treatment was more effective. There was then little knowledge of leukaemogenesis and other stochastic effects of exposure to the accepted therapeutic doses of X-ray radiation. When the technique was first started our fields were limited in apparently early cases to those covering the sacro-iliac joints and the lumbar spine but we found that some patients returned with involvement higher up the spine. The technique was then changed to cover the whole spine in all cases and this technique continued until some doubts arose about possible bone marrow effects.

When the hips, ischial tuberosities, or other joints or muscle attachments were involved, similar treatment was given to the affected part.

There may be marked alleviation of pain and spasm after one or two applications at the beginning of the course of treatment, and by the time the course has finished the majority of patients, if not completely painfree, can rest and sleep naturally. The mental outlook of the patient undergoes a profound change and he becomes more hopeful and confident. He begins to eat properly and to regain weight. As soon as the pain and spasm are diminished active movements were encouraged, particularly breathing exercises to regain mobility of the thorax.

Besides relieving pain and muscle spasm, X-ray treatment also appears to be effective in reducing the activity of the disease. Patients who were pyrexial and cachectic with night sweats become afebrile and convalescent and the disease appears to become quiescent. With such a condition as ankylosing spondylitis, which has remissions and relapses over periods of years, which may proceed to complete ankylosis of the whole spine or which may spontaneously become arrested apparently permanently at any stage of development, it is difficult to assess the long-term effects of a method of treatment.

There are patients who had no sign of recurrence over a period of observation of 20 years and more and I believe that X-ray therapy can render the disease permanently quiescent.

RESULTS

In assessing the results of treatment of the 277 patients previously described, the following criteria were adopted:

In Stage I and Stage II the aim was to restore a symptom-free mobile spine and the results were based on the condition of the whole of the spine.

In Stage III, by definition a large part of the spine is ankylosed. Treatment is directed to relieving pain and spasm and improving the movement of the part of the spine where ankylosis is not complete.

Immediate results within three months of treatment:

Stage I	48 patients	33 symptom-free	68 %
Stage II	181 patients	125 much improved	69 %
Stage III	48 patients	26 much improved	54 %

The long-term follow-up of these patients was not complete and it was possible to make observations on only 106 of the 277 patients after follow-up of 3-5 years. These observations were the following:

		MARKED IMPROVEMENT	
		Symptoms	Signs
Stage I	21 patients	16 (76 %)	Very little loss of movement originally
Stage II	66 patients	48 (72 %)	35 (53 %)
Stage III	19 patients	19 (100 %)	7 (37 %)

Robert Morrison had reported in 1954 that of 164 patients treated, 90 per cent had returned to some sort of work within a year and only 10 per cent had not returned to work.

COMPLICATIONS

Apart from the complications of the disease which have been described, such as iritis which was common in our cases, mitral valvular disease which I have seen only once, an association with ulcerative colitis, and the complications arising from restricted movement, especially of the thorax and the rare one of cervical dislocation, there are some complications and sequelae from irradiation.

Over-irradiation of the skin may cause skin atrophy with telangiectasis and, even later, necrosis in areas where there is rubbing from tight-fitting clothing.

With later knowledge it is obvious that the main hazards are from irradiation of the bone marrow. The treatment described entailed the irradiation of a large proportion of the active bone marrow of the body and we realised that it was necessary to keep a close watch on the peripheral blood count. There were sometimes pronounced leukopenia during treatment which, in some cases, necessitated interruption of treatment. Within a few weeks the blood count returned to normal and, as far as we knew at the time, there were no sequelae.

When there was a report of leukaemia developing in patients treated by X-rays for ankylosing spondylitis and when two such cases were found in my own 1000 cases, we again reduced the area of the spine which was irradiated and gradually also reduced the dose that was given. I was at first confused by the evidence as I had found two cases of previously undiagnosed ankylosing spondylitis among 303 cases of leukaemia treated at the Middlesex Hospital, and wondered if there could be some association between the two diseases.

The technique was altered so that, in addition to routine reduction in the size of the sacro-iliac field and wherever else reduction could be achieved, the skin doses were reduced from 2000 to 1000 rads. I do not know if there has been a discernible alteration in the results achieved in terms of relief of symptoms but working on the tables of Court Brown and Doll's appendix to the 1956 Medical Research Council

Radiosynoviorthesis: local treatment of rheumatoid arthritis

I. Bahous, M.D., Head of the Rheumatological Policlinic of the University of Basel, Switzerland

SUMMARY

Systemic therapy of rheumatoid arthritis is not always satisfactory. If remission occurs it is generally of short duration. Since 1968 the radiosynoviorthesis is a well established local treatment for arthritis. Since more than four years we are using ^{90}Yttrium for the treatment of large joints, ^{186}Rhenium for middle joints, and ^{169}Erbium for small joints. Our results and those in recent literature are very encouraging. Side effects are seldom if the right dosage and the right isotope are used. In the treatment of the knee joint we achieved good or very good results in over 50%. Cases where the therapy has not been successful or very unsatisfactory are joints in an advanced phase of articular destruction and progression of the systemic disease.

Amongst the different procedures for local treatment of chronic synovitis, radiosynoviorthesis became increasingly important during the last few years (1, 3, 5, 6, 8, 10, 11). We have used radioisotopes for the treatment of chronic synovitis in our clinic for the last 4 years, and we have studied effects and side effects of these substances. Today we would like to report on the therapeutic effects of radiosynoviorthesis and histological studies in synovitis.

We have mainly used ^{90}Yttrium which has the best radioactive properties for the treatment of big joints in comparison with other radioisotopes (1, 2, 5). It has an optimal range and does not provide γ-radiation (Tab. I). Its maximal energy of 2.2 MEV is much higher than that of radioactive gold. For the small joints we used ^{169}Erbium which is pre-

TABLE I

Physical Properties of Radio Isotopes

Isotope	Half-life in days	Type of irradiation	Maximal energy in MEV	Tissue penetration in MM Soft tissue Mean value	Tissue penetration in MM Soft tissue Maximal	Tissue penetration in MM Cartilage Mean value	Tissue penetration in MM Cartilage Maximal
169 ER	9,5	β	0,34	0,3	1	0,2	0,7
198 AU	2,7	β γ	0,96 0,41	1,2	3,6	0,9	2,7
186 RE	3,7	β γ little	0,98	1,2	3,7	1	3,1
90 Y	2,7	β	2,2	3,6	11	2,8	8,5

ferred to ^{198}Gold as the latter provides γ-radiation in addition to β-radiation (7). The dosage of the above mentioned radioisotopes was largely determined empirically. As shown in Tab. II we have used radiotherapy in 326 joints with different isotopes. The Table shows that the majority of joints were knee joints. Only a few shoulder and ankle joints received local radiotherapy.

TABLE II

Joints treated (total):	326
Of which	
Knee	210
Hip	17
Ankle	6
Shoulder	16
Elbow	10
Finger	45
Hand	22

Today we only report the results we have obtained with Yttrium in knee joints of patients with rheumatoid arthritis. As shown in Fig. 1 total remission of the local imflammatory process was obtained in 18% of the treated joints by one year, and significant improvement occurred in another 44%. In 30% of the cases no local effect was observed. After 3 years,

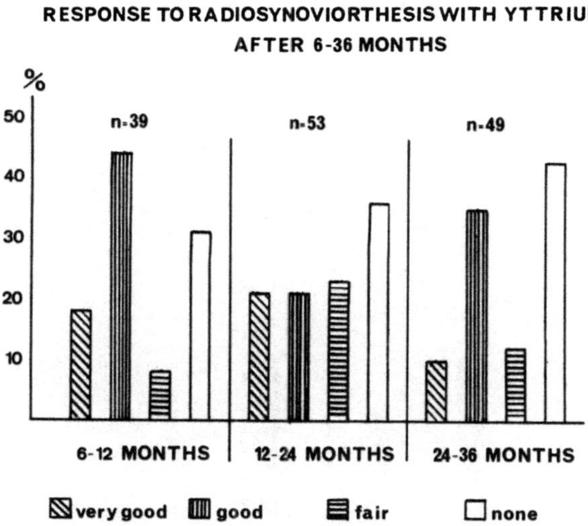

FIGURE 1

Response to radiosynoviorthesis with Yttrium 90 after 6-36 months

only 48% of the knee joints showed good or very good results compared with 62% after one year. Patients who showed no effect received a second injection of Yttrium after 6 months, and again in approximately 50% good or very good results were obtained (Tab. III).

TABLE III

Therapeutic Effect of the Second Yttrium 90 Application 6 Months Following the First Injection

	Improvement		
Number of joints	Good	Fair	None
34	15	13	6

The efficiency of local Yttrium injections is greatly dependent on the stage of the disease and the degree of the local inflammatory process, respectively. Better results were obtained in the early stage of rheumatoid arthritis. In a more advanced stage of the disease radiotherapy was less effective (Fig. 2).

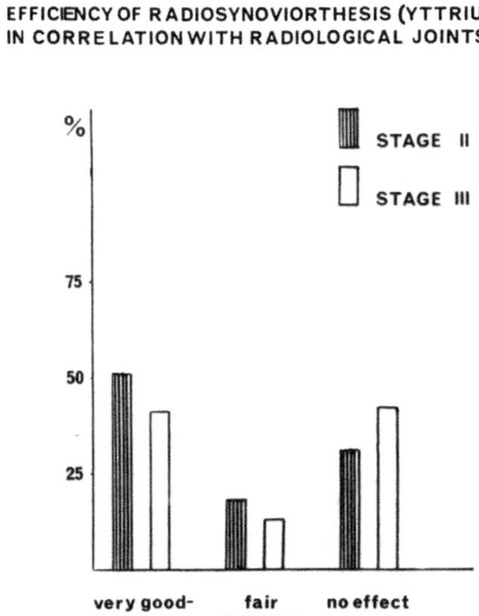

FIGURE 2

Efficiency of radiosynoviorthesis
(Yttrium 90) in Correlation with radiological jointstage

The mode of action of local radiotherapy can partly be explained by the histological changes in the human synovium and by the results of animal experiments. Figure 3 shows a synovitis in rheumatoid arthritis where you notice increased vascularity, hyperplasia of the synovium and heavy cellular infiltrate consisting chiefly of lymphocytes and plasma cells.

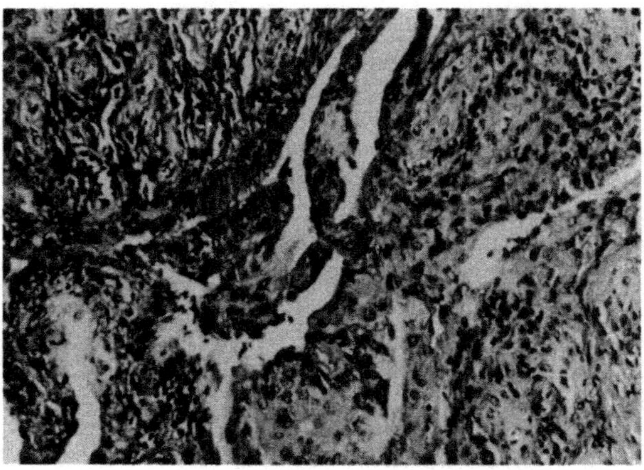

FIGURE 3

Synovitis in rheumatoid arthritis

Three months after intra-articular injection of the radio-isotope the hyperplasia of the synovial lining layers and the cellular infiltration are no longer detectable, and the synovium shows fibrotic changes (Fig. 4).

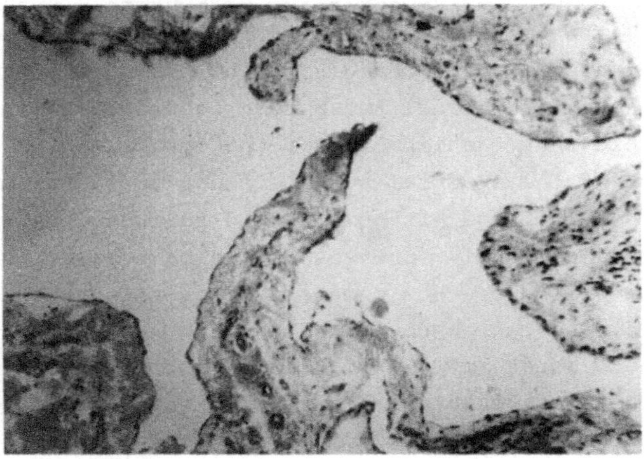

FIGURE 4

Synovitis after treatment with Yttrium 90

It goes without saying that, like for surgical synovectomy, the indications for radiosynoviorthesis have to be strict, since this form of treatment can cause some adverse effects as seen in Tab. IV. During the first days after intra-articular injection of Yttrium local irritations are observed after phagocytosis of the colloidal particles (9, 15). We observed in about 10% of our patients such a radiation synovitis which in general was suppressed effectively with corticosteroids. Occasionally other side effects such as

TABLE IV

Adverse Reactions of Radiosynoviorthesis
Possible
1. General Radiation Reaction
2. Radiation Synovitis
3. Tissue Necrosis
Questionable
1. Early Development of Degenerative Joint Changes
2. Development of Neoplasia
3. Genetic Damage

brief periods of fever, feebleness or lack of appetite were seen. There have been reports of necrosis of inflamed tissues at later time points which was probably related to faulty technique.

As yet nothing is known about the late damages which might occur after intra-articular injection of radionuclids. The observed histological changes in the human synovium and in animal studies equal those seen in old age in man. It is possible that the fibrosis of the synovium with obliteration of the synovial vessels leads to an insufficient supply of the cartilage with oxygen and substrate and tends to premature degenerative changes in the cartilage. Long-term observations will prove how much the cartilaginous tissue is damaged by the radiosynoviorthesis. Further, there is evidence that, after intra-articular injection of radio-isotopes, radioactive material gets into the regional lymph nodes and into the circulation. This causes chromosomal damage in the peripheral lymphocytes (4, 13, 14).

To avoid the local side effects, the following points should be observed: Tab. V injection under sterile conditions, strict intra-articular injection with the help of X-ray control, and pre-injection of a contrasting agent flashing the needle through into the joint space with a corticosteroid suspension to avoid needle track burns. It is also important to observe the dosage guide lines and to use the right isotope. Further, the joints should be immobilized temporarily so as to prevent the radioactive material from leaking from the joint space and to minimize any risk (10, 12).

TABLE V

Provisions for Intraarticular Application of Isotopes

1. **Asepsis**
2. **Strict Intraarticular Injection**
3. **Prevention of Back Flow of Radioactive Material through Injection Canal**
4. **Dosage Guide**
5. **Immobilisation of Joints Following Application**

Comparing advantages and disadvantages of the radiosynoviorthesis in rheumatoid arthritis, we conclude that this form of treatment is most advisable in elderly patients, since the risk of inducing osteoarthritis or neoplasms is small. We believe that in this group of patients radiotherapy is superior to synovectomy, especially when an operation bears certain risks for the patient.

REFERENCES

1. Ansell, B, A. Crook, J.R. Mallard and E.G.L. Bywaters, Evaluation of intra-articular colloidal gold ^{198}Au in the treatment of persistent knee effusions. Ann.Rheum.Dis. 22, 435 (1963).
2. Bridgeman, J.F., F. Bruckner and N.M. Bleehen, Radioactive yttrium in the treatment of rheumatoid knee effusions. Ann.Rheum.Dis. 30, 180 (1971).
3. Bridgeman, J.F., F. Bruckner, V. Eisen, A. Turker and N.M. Bleehen, Irradiation of the synovium in the treatment of rheumatoid arthritis. Quart.J.Med. 166, 357 (1973).
4. De la Chapelle, A, M. Oka, A. Rekonen and A. Ruotsi, Chromosome damage after intra-articular injections of radioactive yttrium. Ann.Rheum.Dis. 31, 508 (1972).
5. Delbarre, F., J. Cayla, C. Menkes, M. Aignan, J-C. Roucayrol and J. Ingrand, La synoviorthèse par les radio-isotopes. La Presse Méd. 76, 1045 (1968).
6. Delbarre, F., J. Cayla, J-C. Roucayrol, C. Menkes, M. Aignan and J. Ingrand, Synoviorthèses (synoviothérapie par les radioisotopes). Etude de plus de 400 traitements et perspectives d'avenir. Ann.Méd. Interne 121, 441 (1970).
7. Delbarre, F., C.J. Menkes, M. Aignan, J. Ingrand and A. Sanchez, Une nouvelle préparation radioactive pour la synoviorthèse: le rhénium 186 colloïdal. Avantages par rapport au colloïde d'or 198. Nouv.Presse Méd. 2, 1372 (1973).

8. Gumpel, J.M., E.D. Williams and H.I. Glass, Use of yttrium 90 in persistent synovitis of the knee. Ann.Rheum.Dis. 32, 223 (1973).
9. Isomäki, A.M., H. Inoue and M. Oka, Uptake of ^{90}Y resin colloid by synovial fluid cells and synovial membrane in rheumatoid arthritis. Scand.J.Rheum. 1, 53 (1972).
10. Oka, M., A. Rekonen, A. Ruotsi and O. Seppälä, Intra-articular injection of Y-90-resin colloid in the treatment of rheumatoid knee joint effusions. Acta Rheum. Scand. 17, 148 (1971).
11. Prichard, H.L., J.F. Bridgeman and N.M. Bleehen, An investigation of radioactive yttrium (90Y) for the treatment of chronic knee effusions. Br.J.Radiol. 43, 466 (1970).
12. Rekonen, A., M. Oka and A. Ruotsi, Intra-articularly injected 90Y resin colloid: Distribution fate and dosimetry. Rheumatologie 2: Suppl. 1, 57 (1972).
13. Stevenson, A.C., Chromosomal damage in human lymphocytes from radio-isotope therapy. Ann.Rheum.Dis. 32, Suppl. 6, 19 (1973).
14. Stevenson, A.C., J. Bedford, G.W. Dolphin, R.J. Purrott, D.C. LLoyd, A.G.S. Hill, H.F.H. Hill, J.M. Gumpel, D. Williams, J.T. Scott, N.W. Ramsey, F.E. Bruckner and C.B.D.A. Fearn, Cytogenetic and scanning study of patients receiving intra-articular injections of gold-198 and yttrium-90. Ann.Rheum.Dis. 32, 112 (1973).
15. Webb, F.W.S., J. Lowe and R. Bluestone, Uptake of colloidal radioactive yttrium by synovial membrane. Ann.Rheum.Dis. 28, 300 (1969).

Comparison of the efficacy of ^{224}Ra and other radio-isotopes in the treatment of rheumatoid arthritis

A. Bertrand, J. Martin and C. Hocquard
Service de Médecine Nucléaire C.H.U. Brabois 54500 Vandoeuvre

ABSTRACT

In the course of chronic inflammation rheumatism, synovial inflammation plays a major role in the production of osteo-cartilaginous lesions. The aim of different therapeutics is to destroy this pathological articular tissue. The use of radio-isotope in the treatment of chronic synovial effusion has been proposed since 1968. The authors compare the characteristics and the results of the ^{224}Ra with four other radio-isotopes.

For several years, one of the objects of local treatment of rheumatoid arthritis has been to destroy the hypertrophy of the synovial membrane or panus, the latter behaving like a tumour tissue which tends to invade gradually the structures composing the joint.

To counteract this proliferation, surgical synovectomy has been proposed since 1930. It has generally given good results, but the risks are not always null and the general and local contra-indications often prevent operation. Furthermore, certain joints such as the hip, are not very suitable for this operation.

Thus, certain physicians propose medical synovectomy by local injection of sclerosing substances, such as osmic acid, but the results are, on the whole, mediocre and very variable.

It was thus decided to use the action of ionising radiation and to carry out intra-articular injection of a radio-isotope. Colloidal ^{198}Gold was the first one used, but owing to relatively high energy gamma radiation, other radioactive substances, such as ^{169}Erbium, ^{90}Yttrium and ^{186}Rhenium were proposed. Owing to the good results obtained with ^{224}Ra in the treatment of ankylosing spondylitis, certain rheumatologists also use it for these intra-articular injections. Other isotopes were used, but for too short a period to be mentioned here.

The success of this treatment used throughout the world in thousands of patients, no longer requires proof, but it has not always been easy to choose the radio-isotope. With now more than 10 years follow-up it appears that certain radio-isotopes should be banned and others only used in special cases.

CHARACTERISTICS OF THE FIVE RADIO-ISOTOPES

Although all these 5 radio-isotopes have roughly similar physical periods, from 2.6 to 9.4 days, the various types of emission are extremely variable. It appears that these 5 radio-isotopes all emit beta rays. These electrons are responsible for the local therapeutic effect obtained in synoviortheses. Only ^{224}Ra is an alpha emitter. The 5 radio-isotopes are also all gamma emitters but in very variable proportions. Thus, Erbium with photons, the energy of which is only 0.008 MEV, and Yttrium which emits photons at 0.75 MEV have only 0.02% emission, and should not be considered as important gamma emitters.

^{224}Ra may thus be differentiated from other radio-elements by this alpha emission: these particles have only a very short course in the soft tissues, about a few tenths of a micron, their course is rectilinear. Along these few microns, several MEV are dissipated in collision with molecules which constitute the medium. The effect of the alpha particles is thus superficial but very brutal. Furthermore, the radio-

TABLE I

KIND OF RADIATION

	Half life	Alpha	Beta	Gamma	Maximum range of beta particles in soft tissue
RADIUM 224 and his daughters	3,64 days	yes	yes	yes	12 mm
YTTRIUM 90	2,6 days	no	yes	rare	11 mm
GOLD 198	2,7 days	no	yes	yes	3,6 mm
ERBIUM 169	9,4 days	no	yes	rare	1 mm
RHENIUM 186	3,7 days	no	yes	rare	3,7 mm

TABLE II

KIND OF RADIATION (ENERGY : MEV)

	Alpha particles	Beta particles	Gamma rays
RADIUM 224 and his daughters	5,68 (95 %) 5,44 (5 %) 6,28 (99 %) 5,74 (0,3 %) 6,78 (100 %) 6,02 (35 %) 8,78 (85 %)	0,34 (84 %) 0,58 (12 %) 1,80 (47 %) 1,02 (35 %) 2,38 (35 %) 2,25 (65 %)	The most important are : 0,239 (84 %) 0,300 (100 %) 0,115 (100 %) 0,410 (100 %) 0,162 (65 %) 0,124 (65 %) 2,20 (65 %) 2,61 (35 %)
YTTRIUM 90	-	2,27 (100 %)	1,75 (0,02 %)
GOLD 198	-	0,96 (99 %) 0,28 (1 %) 1,37 (0,02 %)	0,412 (99 %) 0,690 (1 %) 1,090 (2 %)
ERBIUM 169	-	0,340 (58 %)	0,008 (42 %)
RHENIUM 186	-	1,07 (73 %) 0,96 (23 %)	0,137 (23 %) 0,123 (2 %) 0,630 (0,2 %) 0,770 (0,3 %)

biological effects of these heavy particles are ill-known. Thus, may be doubted the utility of such rays in synoviorthesis.

Beta rays have a much higher penetration as, on average, the course varies between 1 and 11 mm, the quantity of energy liberated during the various collisions, is only a few tenths of a MEV and their course is very sinuous. It therefore results that the biological effect of beta rays is better distributed in depth and less brutal.

Gamma rays are generally parasitic rays for, owing to their very high penetrating power, the energy liberated locally is very low. Their only interest is the possibility of carrying out satisfactory arthro-scintigraphy in order to ensure that the injected product is well within the joint.

From this short analysis it appears that only beta emissions seem to have a positive effect in synoviorthesis and that alpha and gamma rays are of little interest, except perhaps, that gamma rays may produce arthro-scintiscans.

TABLE III

	PHYSICAL and CHEMICAL STATE	QUANTITY ADMINISTERED PER JOINT	CRITIC ORGANS
RADIUM 224	Aqueous solution of radium chloride	28 to 84 microcuries	Skeleton
YTTRIUM 90	Colloidal particle of yttrium citrate Size 100 Å	3 to 6 millicuries	Lymph nodes
GOLD 198	Colloid of gold stabilized with gelatin Size 200 - 400 Å	3 to 6 millicuries	Lymph nodes
ERBIUM 169	Colloidal particle of erbium citrate Size 100 Å	0,25 to 1 millicurie	Lymph nodes
RHENIUM 180	Colloidal particle of rhenium sulfure Size 100 Å	3 to 6 millicuries	Lymph nodes

Analysis of Table III shows the fundamental difference in their physio-chemical form of their therapeutic use for these 5 radio-elements. Only ^{224}Ra is presented in aqueous solution in the form of a chloride. On the other hand, the other 4 radio-elements, are all colloids, the diameter of which varies between 100 and 400 Angstrom. We have carried out a study on the elimination of radium chloride after injection into the joint of knees of several patients. The results show that the fall in activity of ^{224}Ra and its by-products occurred approximately according to two exponential curves: 60 to 80% with a short half life of about 1 hour and 20 to 40% with a longer half life of 11 hours. ^{224}Ra leaves the joint cavity passing into the blood and is deposited on the whole skeleton and soft tissues, where it is eliminated into the urine and stools.

On the other hand, the other radio-isotopes commercialised in the form of colloids stay in the joint cavity for a much longer period. These colloid particles are eliminated by the lymphatic system and after injection into the knee, for example, it is mainly in the inguinal and pelvic lymph nodes that they are found.

Table IV shows that the size of these particles plays an important role but that the migrating activities are relatively low compared with those of ^{224}Ra, as, only in 30% of cases, is more than 2% of the injected activity found in the pelvis.

TABLE IV

RELATION BETWEEN THE SIZE OF COLLOIDS
AND THE ACTIVITY OF LYMPHATIC MIGRATION (J. INGRAND)

AUTHORS		SIZE OF COLLCID	NUMBER OF CASE WITH IMPORTANT MIGRATION (⩾ 2 %)
VIRRKUNEN	Au 198	200 A	32/90
TOPP	"	300 A	4/18
ROUCAYROL, DELBARRE	"	300 A	4/21
MAKIN	"	700 A	-
CORRENS	"	3000 A	nul
DELBARRE et ROUCAYROL	Y 90 Er 169	Heterogeneous 1-10 60 % 10-1000 30 % 1000 10 %	11/37

It may be concluded from the latter that only radio-isotopes prepared in the form of colloids should be used in this form of treatment.

INJECTED QUANTITIES

Analysis of the quantities injected per joint shows relatively marked differences depending of the radio-isotopes. Thus, for ^{224}, the injected doses relatively low, a few tenths of a microcurie. On the other hand, in the case of Yttrium, gold and Rhenium the activity was about one millicurie. In the case of Erbium, the injected quantities were lower for this radio-isotope emits low energy electrons. It is mainly used for small joints such as interphalangeal joints. In view of their small volume, the quantities injected within the joint are limited to a few tenths of a millicurie.

DOSIMETRY

High doses are delivered to the joints. This is appropriate since the destruction of pannus is directly related to the quantity of radioactivity present. In the case of gold, Rhenium and Yttrium, and for activities varying between 3 and 6 millicuries, most authors consider the dose delivered about 5 to 10,000 rads per joint. In the case of ^{224}Ra, there is no precise date. On the contrary, for the remainder of the organism, the information seems more complete. For colloids, the target organs are mainly the lymph nodes and, according to Rekonen's work, the doses delivered at the level of the inguinal lymph nodes vary between 300 and 500 rads after intra-articular injection into the knee of 5 millicuries of Yttrium. In view of the physical characteristics of the other radio-isotopes, the doses for the other colloids should be of the same order. For ^{224}Ra, the target organ is the skeleton and, according to the work of Schales and Mayes, the average doses delivered to the skeleton are about 0.2 rads per microcurie. Thus for an injection of 84 microcuries, the dose delivered to the skeleton is about 20 rads. But if several joints are treated simultaneously, this value increases in proportion.

CLINICAL RESULTS

Table V summarizes all the results obtained with ^{224}Ra, ^{90}Yttrium, ^{186}Rhenium and ^{169}Erbium in Nacy and with ^{198}Gold in Paris (Pr. Roucayrol).

It appears that on the whole these 5 radio-isotopes give relatively good results, the 4 presented in the form of a colloid seem to have greater efficacy than ^{224}Ra. According to Tables I, II and III, one may expect this finding.

TABLE V

RESULTS OF ISOTOPIC SYNOVIORTHESIS

	RADIUM 224 (Nancy)	YTTRIUM 90 (Nancy)	GOLD 198 (Roucayrol Paris)	RHENIUM 186 (Nancy)	ERBIUM 169 (Nancy)
Number of synoviorthesis	180	152	-	20	108
Good results	35 %	63 %	69 %	70 %	72 %
Incompleted improvement	38 %	27 %	25 %	25 %	18 %
Absence of improvement	27 %	10 %	11 %	10 %	10 %

CONCLUSIONS

In view of the physical and physicochemical characteristics of solutions of ^{224}Radium chloride, and furthermore, the very average results obtained, this radio-isotope should no longer be used in synoviorthesis. Colloidal gold, owing to the gamma radiation, should also be avoided. ^{90}Yttrium and ^{186}Rhenium should be used for the large joints and ^{169}Erbium, owing to its low energy beta radiation, should be reserved for the metacarpal and inter-phalangeal joints.

REFERENCES

1. Roucayrol, J.C., Introduction à la biophysique de la synoviorthèse par les isotopes bêta émetteurs. Rhumatologie 19-23 (1972).
2. Ingrand, J., Les éléments de choix d'une préparation radioactive destinée à la synoviorthèse. Rhumatologie 25-31 (1972).
3. Menkes, C-J., M. Dignan et B. Galmiche, Le traitement des rhumatismes par les synoviorthèses. Rhumatologie 61-80 (1972).
4. Rekonen, A., M. Oka and A. Ruotsi, Intra-articulary injected ^{90}Y resin colloid: distribution, fate and

dosimetry. R.Bull.Lig.Internat.Rhum. à paraître.
5. Spiess, Heinz and Charles W. Mayes, Bone cancers induced by ^{224}Ra (ThX). In: Children and Adult, Health Physics Pergamon Press Vol. 19 (1970) 713-729.

Experimental data on the injection of ^{224}Ra into the kneejoint of rats and rabbits*

B. Wallner and W.A. Müller
Institut für Biologie Gesellschaft für Strahlen- und Umweltforschung mbH D-8042 Neuherberg/Federal Republic of Germany

ABSTRACT

The distribution of ^{224}Ra in rats was studied after intra-articular injections. The autoradiographic results and the measurements of activity of bone and soft tussue were compared with corresponding data obtained after i.v.- and i.p.-injections.

In addition the distribution pattern of ^{224}Ra after intra-articular injections into the knee-joints of untreated rabbits and of rabbits after experimental induction of arthritis was studied.

INTRODUCTION

^{224}Ra is used in the therapy of arthritis in human patients since about 10 years (1). In order to estimate the possible risk of late effects in these patients we studied the distribution of ^{224}Ra after intra-articular application in healthy young rats and rabbits. In addition preliminary data on rabbits with experimental arthritis are presented.

* In association with EURATOM (Contract No. 218-76-1 BIO D).

MATERIALS AND METHODS

Experiments with rats: Female Wistar-Neuherberg rats, 6 months old, received one single injection of 5 μCi ^{224}Ra as chloride in isotonic solution into one knee-joint. Before the injection the animals were anaesthetized with a 2% solution of Evipan-Natrium i.p..

2 h, 24 h, 48 h and 7 days after injection each 5 animals were sacrificed. The animals were used for physical measurement of the activity of ^{224}Ra and its daughter product ^{212}Pb in both knee-joints, femur, thoracic vertebra, kidneys, spleen and liver and for autoradiographic studies of both knee-joints, thoracic vertebra, kidneys, spleen and liver. The knee-joint sample included the cartilage and the connective tissue of the joint, the distal and proximal part of femur and tibia with the metaphyseal region. Measurement of radioactivity was performed with a well-type-crystal (NaI). For autoradiography the knee-joints and the thoracic vertebrae were embedded in methacrylate (2) after fixation and dehydration in alcohol for 27 hours.

Experiments with rabbits: Rabbits, a half year old, with a weight of 2-3 kg received s.c. 4 ccm of bovine-albumine (30%). After twenty days 0.1-0.2 ccm of this albumine was injected each day into the knee-joints for fourteen days (3).

The rabbits were divided into two groups: The animals of the first group received 20 μCi ^{224}Ra in one knee-joint one day after the last injection of albumine and were killed one day and three weeks after the incorporation of ^{224}Ra. The second group served as control for observation of the untreated arthritis.

In addition two healthy rabbits received 20 μCi ^{224}Ra in one knee-joint, and were also killed one day and three weeks after the injection of the radionuclide.

The joint-capsules were prepared plus the synovial membranes, embedded into methacrylate and autoradiographies were made of those treated with ^{224}Ra. The distribution was determined with measurements of radioactivity in the same way as at the rats.

RESULTS AND DISCUSSION

Figure 1 shows the distribution in per cent of the intra-articulary injected activity in the skeleton and different organs. The values are corrected for the physical half-life. The activity in cpm on the ordinate is plotted on a logarithmic scale; the abscissa shows the days after the incorporation.

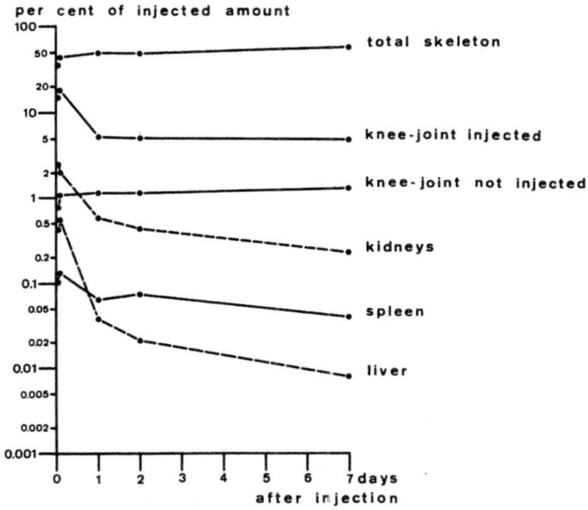

FIGURE 1

Distribution of intra-articulary injected ^{224}Ra in the organism of the rat

Already after two hours 50% of the injected ^{224}Ra is found in the total skeleton. Only 5% of the injected activity remained in the injected joint twenty-four hours after the incorporation with a rapid decrease of the initial activity. Kidney, liver and spleen contain only fractions of one per cent of the total activity after twenty-four hours.

Figure 2 shows the dose rate in rad/day, based on *one* μCi ^{224}Ra injected into the knee-joint. The number above the curves indicate total mean doses of the respective organs. We find the greatest dose burden at the point of injection. The not-injected knee shows the same dose efficiency as the total skeleton (maximum 15-20 rad/day). The

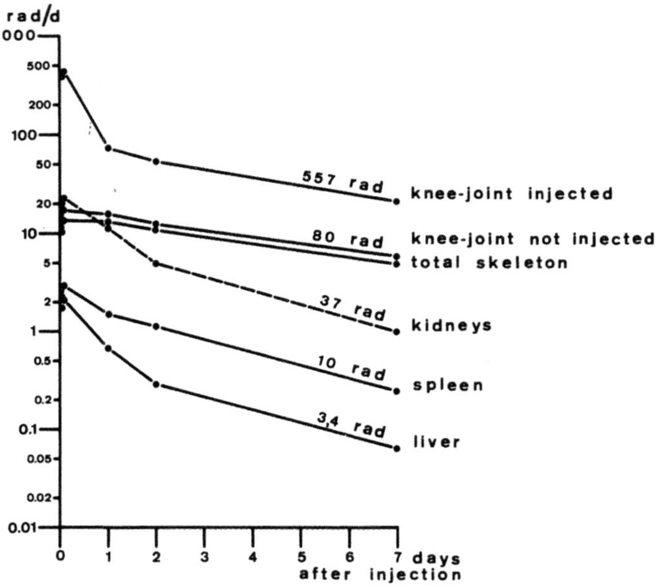

FIGURE 2

Dose burden of total skeleton, knee-joints, kidney, spleen and liver of the rat after intra-articular injection of 1 μCi ^{224}Ra

kidney as excretive organ initially has a somewhat higher dose efficiency, while liver and spleen show only 12% and 4% respectively of the burden of the skeleton.

For comparison we studied the distribution pattern after i.v.-injections of ^{224}Ra. Apart from the knee-joint, the distribution pattern and the radiation burden is very similar as after intra-artcular injections. In previous experiments the distribution was studied after i.p.-injection ^{224}Ra in rats with nearly identical results (4).

Figure 3 shows an autoradiographic picture of the proximal end of the tibia with the joint cartilage, two hours after intra-articular incorporation. A strong concentration of activity is seen at the border line between joint cartilage and the articular surface of the bone.

Figure 4 shows the growth zone of the tibia of the non-injected knee-joint, two hours after the intra-articular injection. We find the usual picture with the highest con-

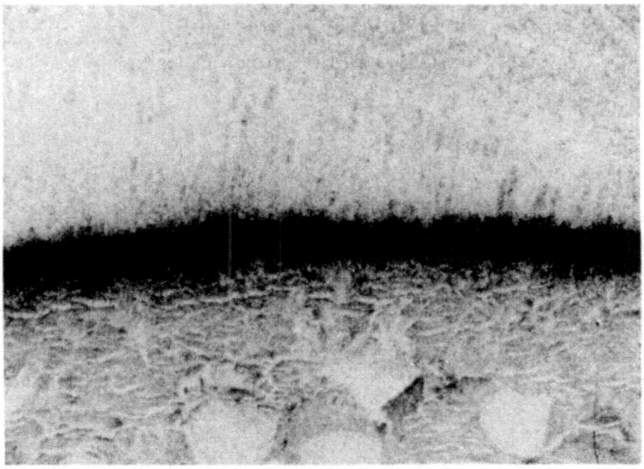

FIGURE 3

Autoradiography of the proximal end of the tibia with the joint-cartilage, two hours after intra-articular incorporation

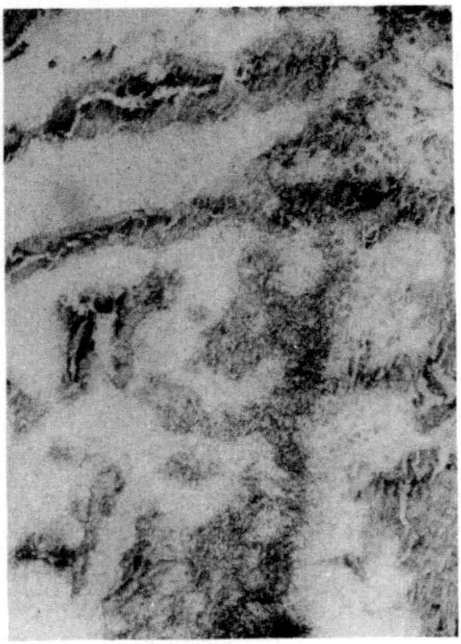

FIGURE 4

Autoradiography of the growth area of the tibia of the non-injected knee-joint, two hours after the intra-articular injection

centration of activity in the area of calcification of cartilage and primary spongiosa.

In the autoradiographies of the thoracic vertebrae tracks can be clearly seen on the bone surfaces two hours after the intra-articular injections.

After 24 and 48 hours and 7 days after the incorporation, we find a low density of tracks at the border line between joint cartilage and the articular surface of the bone as it is shown in Figure 5.

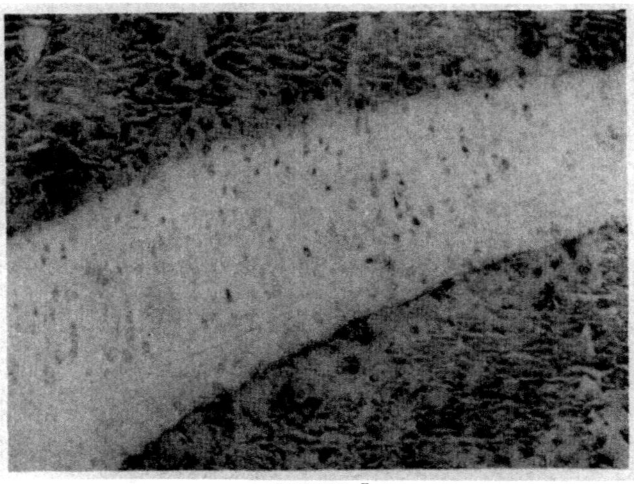

FIGURE 5

Autoradiography of the proximal end of the tibia with the joint-cartilage, seven days after intra-articular incorporation

From the data demonstrated one can state, that also the autoradiographies of ^{224}Ra after intra-articular injections into the knee-joints of healthy rats rather similar to those after i.v.- and i.p.-injections.

Figure 6 shows the distribution of ^{224}Ra itself and its daughter product ^{212}Pb twenty-four hours after injection of 20 µCi ^{224}Ra into the knee-joint of an arthritic animal (*above*) and an untreated one (*below*). In all *soft* tissue organs a surplus of the daughter ^{212}Pb can be observed - this is the same as in untreated rats - as shown in Figure 7.

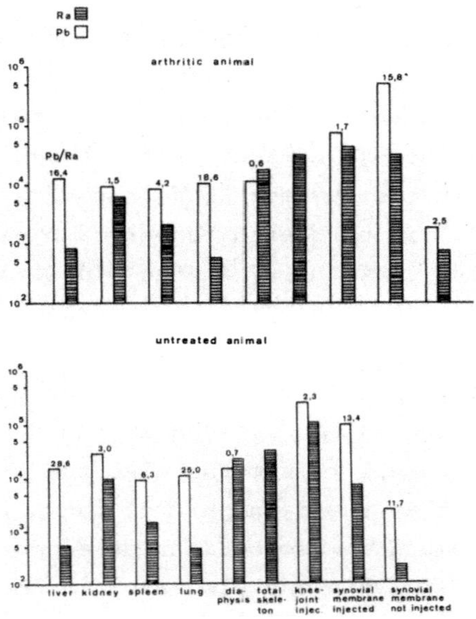

FIGURE 6

Distribution of ^{224}Ra and ^{212}Pb (per gram fresh organ weight) 24 hours after intra-articular injection of ^{224}Ra into the knee-joint of the rabbit

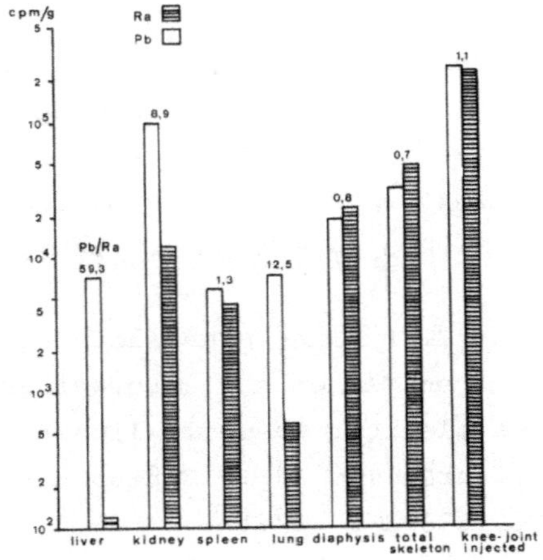

FIGURE 7

Distribution of ^{224}Ra and ^{212}Pb (per gram fresh organ weight) 24 hours after intra-articular injection of ^{224}Ra into the knee-joint of the untreated rat

The same phenomenon is normal also after i.p.- and i.v.-injections.

But the extent of this ^{212}Pb-surplus is remarkable especially in the knee-joint-area. Here values of the Pb/Ra ratio - as given in the numbers above the bars - between 1.1 in rats and 2.3 in untreated rabbits can be observed. The arthritic value is with 1.7 in the middle. But if one considers the ratio for the synovial membrane in the rabbits, an excessive high surplus of ^{212}Pb, that is to say 15 times more ^{212}Pb-activity than ^{224}Ra, can be seen. Even the highest absolute ^{212}Pb-concentration is seen in the synovial membrane of the arthritic animal, this means also the highest dose rate and suggests that the main part of radiation effects on the synovial membrane must be attributed more to ^{212}Pb than to ^{224}Ra itself. This may also explain the missing of tracks in the autoradiographies of the synovial membranes because due to the short half-life of 10.6 hours of ^{212}Pb the tracks could not be present nearly one week after sacrifice, the time which was necessary for embedding and exposition.

REFERENCES

1. Louyot, P., Y. Laurent-Montet, J. Bertrand, B. Legras, J. Stines and J. Pourel, Résultats de la synoviothérapie par le Radium 224. In: Les synoviorthèses dans le traitement des Maladies Rhumatismales (M. Aignan and M. Douis, Eds.), pp. 125-141. Paris, May 26-27 (1971).
2. Hinderinger, B. and G. Büsing, Schnelleinbettung unentkalkter Knochen von Mäusen für autoradiographische Untersuchungen kurzlebiger wasserlöslicher Isotope durch ein Kontaktverfahren mit AR 10 Strippingfilm. Histochemie 26, 333-342 (1971).
3. Klinge, F. Beitr. Path.Anat. 83, 185 (1929/30).
4. Müller, W.A., Studies on short-lived internal α-emitters in mice and rats. Part I. ^{224}Ra. Int.J.Radiat.Biol. 20, 27-38 (1971).

Intravenous injection of ^{224}Ra in morbus Paget

W. Koch, Dr.med. Professor of the Orthopaedic Clinic of the University Münster/Westfalen, Federal Republic of Germany

SUMMARY

Since 1957 we have treated 21 patients with Morbus Paget and monostotic or polyostotic involvement of the skeleton with ^{224}Ra. The radiobiological effect of low-dosage ^{224}Ra with weekly injections of 2.8 μCi and a total of 12 injections alleviates pain and helps to stabilize the Paget bone by increasing the bone sclerosis and prohibiting the expansion of the granulation tissue. A progression or reappearance of Paget lesions was not to be avoided in each case and ^{224}Ra therapy had to be repeated in 8 patients. Therefore annual clinical and roentgenographic examinations of the Paget patients are indicated. To verify the diagnosis and to exclude sarcomatoid degeneration a biopsy should be performed before the therapy with ^{224}Ra is started.

The etiology and largely also the pathogenesis of Morbus Paget are still obscure. Henschen alone mentions 15 different theories, of which the chronic inflammation and disorders of vascularisation are of etiological importance. Süss examined the pathologically increased vascularisation of the Paget bone angiographically and decided that venous valve atrophy in the bone is responsible for the osteitis deformans. Already about 90 years ago Paget suspected a pathogenesis of inflammation, which was the reason for Hellner to adhere to the name of osteitis deformans, although he does not exclude the possibility of constitutional factors. Jones and Reed surmise that there is a dominant autosomal hereditary factor, and according to Steinbach 3.5 per cent of the total population above 45 years are afflicted by the disease.

Considering the obscure etiology and pathogenesis of Morbus Paget, it is not surprising that we have no causal therapy as yet. There is a wide range of therapeutic measures including analgesics, antiinflammatory drugs, sex hormones, as well as the rather problematic treatment with cytostatics. Maurer maintains that the antiinflammatory radiation treatment only eases the subjective symptomes but does not influence the process of the disease itself. Parenteral radiotherapy with radioactive phosphor P^{32} also induces only pain relief, according to Axler. In 1952, Mahlo reported on the positive effect of oral ^{224}Ra treatment in 6 patients. Koch, in 1957, recommended i.v. low-dosage application of ^{224}Ra in Morbus Paget with an average of 12 injections of 2.8 μCi at weekly intervals. This dosage which is 10 times lower than that used for i.v. ^{224}Ra treatment in spondylitis

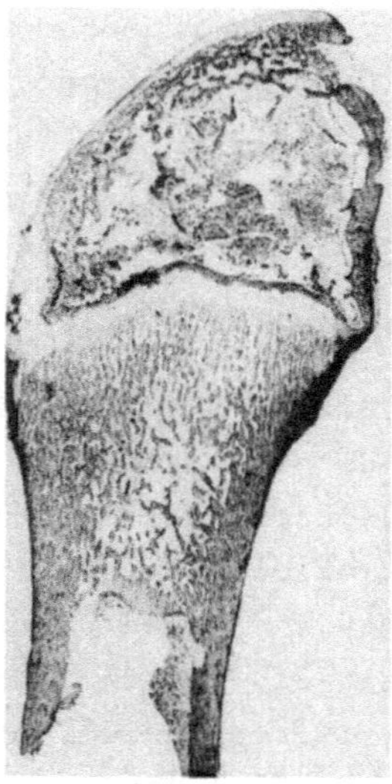

FIGURE 1

Spongiosclerosis of the distal femoral epiphysis of the rabbit after low-dosage ^{224}Ra application

ankylopoetica, induces spongiosclerosis, as we demonstrated by experimental tests (Fig. 1). Osteoclast activity is reduced while the function of the osteoblasts remains normal. Beta- and gamma-radiation of the disintegration products of ^{224}Ra stops the progress of the vascular granulation tissue in the Paget bone, thereby stimulating the osteoblast activity, and this entails a normalization and solidification of the bone structures while the pains due to periost stretching and laceration in the Paget bone are alleviated.

Between 1956 and 1973 we have treated 21 patients with histologically verified Morbus Paget at our hospital, 5 of them with monostotic affliction of the skeleton, in 16 the disease was polyostotic. The most common sites of Paget lesions were in the pelvis, vertebral body, femur, and skull, corresponding to the distribution mentioned by Schmorl. We had 10 male and 11 female patients, while according to Schmorl the male representation is slightly predominant with 58 per cent. Our youngest patient was 18 years old; the majority was between 50 and 60 years old, which agrees with the data reported by Kienböck who found the onset of Morbus Paget to be at an age between 40 and 60, and at the earliest after puberty. At the last follow-up examination 3 out 14 patients had died after cardiovascular complications, 1 patient after an accident and another due to tumor metastasis of the prostate.

Evaluation of the roentgenograms shows a progressive density of the bone structures in the left iliac bone and acetabulum in a 59-year old man 4 years after i.v. ^{224}Ra therapy with 15 injections of 2.8 μCi. Thus a protrusio acetabuli was avoided which is a rather common feature in Morbus Paget (Fig. 2).
In spite of 2 therapeutic attempts with ^{224}Ra at an interval of 3 years, this 57-year old patient developed a leftsided coxarthrosis 5 years after the onset of Morbus Paget with involvement of the left pelvis. Painful ankylosis of the hip necessitated the implantation of an artificial hip joint (Fig. 3).

A particularly favourable course of the disease was seen

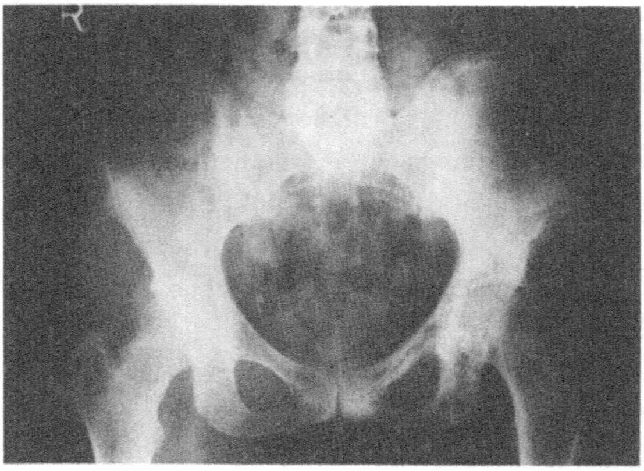

FIGURE 2

Increased spongiosclerosis of the left pelvis and acetabulum in a 59-year old man 4 years after ^{224}Ra treatment

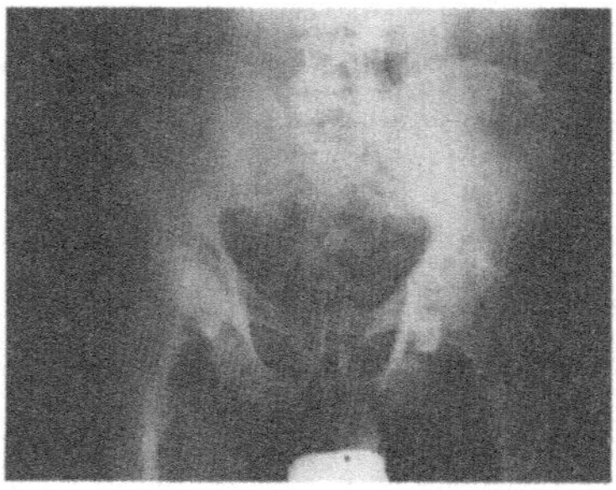

FIGURE 3

5 Years after the onset of Morbus Paget a coxarthrosis developed in this 57-year old patient in spite of 2 therapeutic attempts with ^{224}Ra

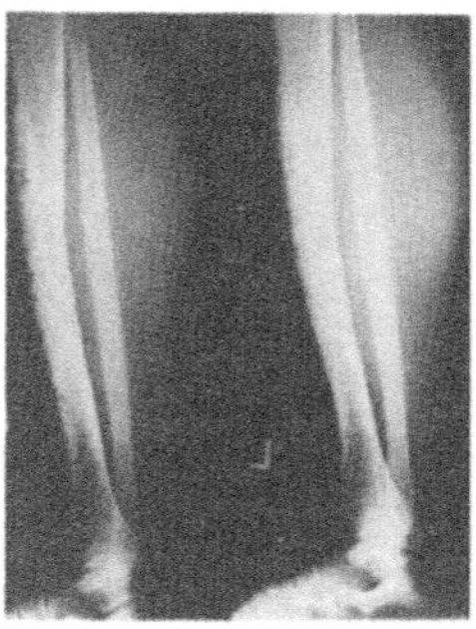

FIGURE 4

5 Years after ^{224}Ra treatment spongiosclerosis (on the right side in the picture) increased in the left tibia of a 25-year old woman with monostotic affliction

in a 25-year old nurse with monostotic affliction of the left tibia (Fig. 4). After 2 series of ^{224}therapy at an interval of 2 years with 10 injections of 2.8 μCi each, a marked increase of sclerosis was seen in the Paget bone 5 years after the last injection. The usual expansion of the focal Paget lesions and the increased tibia bowing which is often seen in association with cortex fissures did not occur.

Contrary to this, the disease progressed in a 67-year old patient with monostotic involvement of the tibia. 11 Years after a single series of 20 injections of 2.8 μCi the focal lesions had expanded and a transformation zone at the tibial head was noticeable together with slightly increased antecurvation (Fig. 5).

This case history demonstrates clearly that all Morbus Paget patients treated with ^{224}Ra should be reexamined at annual intervals so that a second series of ^{224}Ra could be administered if indicated by the clinical and roentgenographic results. We thought this necessary in 8 cases of our group. This practice may help to inhibit the recurrence of bone pain caused by the progression or regeneration of Paget lesions and give hope of a remission particularly in polyostotic cases. Such considerations should have been applied in the case of a female patient, aged 54, who got 14 injections of ^{224}Ra of 2.8 μCi; without noticeable symptoms it came to a progression of the disease during the following 12 years, involving the total humerus with severe antecurvation, although without infraction (Fig. 6).

Of course it does not necessarily come to an expansion of the Paget lesions after a single series of ^{224}Ra therapy, as finally demonstrated by the increasing bone sclerosis in a monostotic inflected collar-bone of a 75-year old woman 8 years after 10 injections of ^{224}Ra of 2.8 μCi (Fig. 7).

Summarizing one can say about the radiobiological effect of ^{224}Ra and its disintegration products in Morbus Paget that it induces a sclerosis of the Paget bone by disturbing the osteoclast activity and simultaneously stimulating the osteoblast function, while the proliferation of the

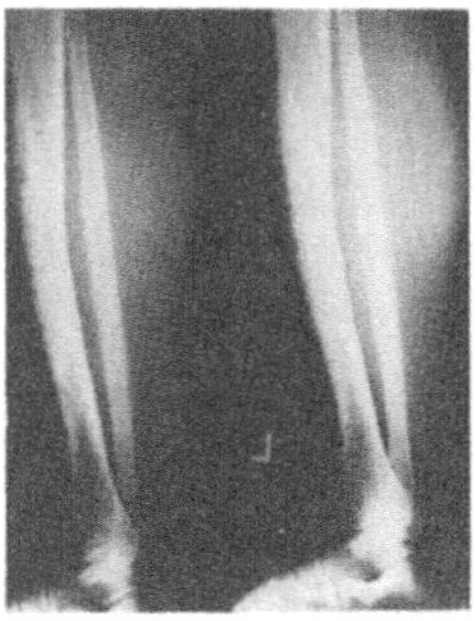

FIGURE 5

11 Years after ^{224}Ra therapy the Paget lesions increased in the tibia of a 67-year old man

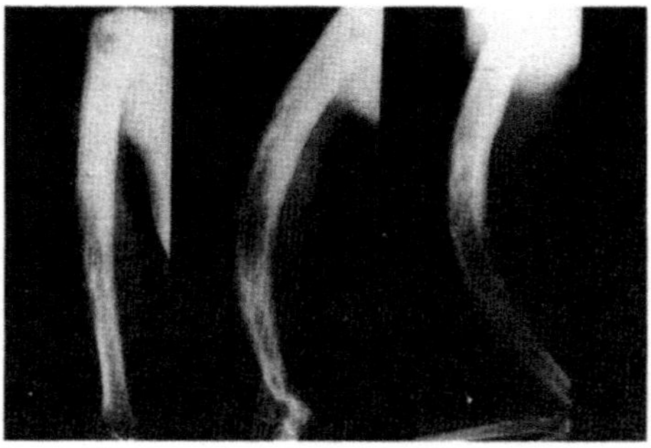

FIGURE 6

Increase of Paget lesions and antecurvation of the humerus in a 54-year old woman 12 years after ^{224}Ra treatment

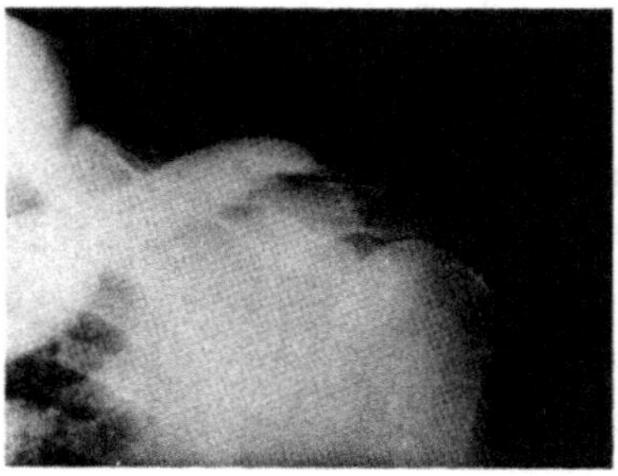

FIGURE 7

Increasing bone sclerosis in a monostotic inflected collar-bone of a 75-year old woman 8 years after ^{224}Ra therapy osteolytic vascular granulation tissue is prohibited. Thus the affected tubular bone of the lower limbs is more adaptable to statical and functional stress and severe deformation and fracturing are inhibited. A progression or new appearance of Paget lesions cannot be excluded after a single series of ^{224}Ra injections. Therefore annual clinical and roentgenographic reexamination of the Paget patients is mandatory in order to decide upon the necessity of a repeated ^{224}Ra treatment.

In none of our Morbus Paget patients treated with low-dosage ^{224}Ra we saw an immediate or late impairment of the haematogenic or parenchymal organs. Before the ^{224}Ra treatment is initiated, a biopsy should be performed in order to verify the diagnosis and to exclude a possible sarcoma, as we saw it in a 70-year old patient at our hospital.

According to our experiences the treatment of Morbus Paget with ^{224}Ra is a valuable method which should be tried more extensively in a larger number of patients.

Literature on request from the author.

Clinical experiences concerning late effects and risks of ^{224}Ra

H. Spiess, Dr.med. Professor
Kinderpoliklinik der Universität München, D-8000,
Federal Republic of Germany

Introducing my talk, I like to give some details from the history of our study.

When I was asked at the beginning of 1948 to test a new drug against tuberculosis, I was an assistant of the University Children's Hospital at Göttingen and in charge of the tuberculosis ward. At this time we were engaged in experimental tuberculosis. And at this time I had already some experience with Streptomycin, which had saved the lives of some of our patients with generalized tuberculosis. This was the reason I was asked to test the new drug called Peteosthor which was used by Dr. Troch against tuberculosis, ankylosing spondylitis and other diseases.

We asked him as initiator of this mixture of ^{224}Ra and Platinum-Eosin-dye to send us some amount of Peteosthor for bacteriological, experimental and clinical testing. He refused because it should be tested exclusively under his supervision. So my boss at this time, who was Dean of the faculty of medicine, urged me to go for one year to Hildesheim where the Insurance-Company of Brunswick (Landesversicherungsanstalt Braunschweig) had a small hospital (Trillkegut) very well equipped for the Peteosthor-treatment of patients and the laboratory and animal experiments. Some other collegues came from University Hospitals at Göttingen, Heidelberg and Münster.

Consequently the first we did was to test the potency

of Peteosthor bacteriologically in vitro, second to test it in animal experiments in view of the potency against tuberculosis and the hypothesis of Dr. Troch (10). The first results in vitro and the animal tests on the distribution of ^{224}Ra with or without Platinum and the Eosin dye we got already after some weeks before the end of the year 1948.

My first rabbit experiment could not confirm Dr. Troch's hypothesis that ^{224}Ra is guided to the sick bone tissue if it is injected intravenously in the mixture of Peteosthor.

After 4 weeks I told Dr. Troch, that ^{224}Ra is deposited mainly in the growing bone, irrespective of its being injected with or without Platinum-Eosin addition.

The result of this communication was the locking of the doors of my animal laboratory. I had to continue our animal experiments in Göttingen. The first 2 papers about our own experimental data were published in 1950 (1, 2). With Tietz we could show that ^{224}Ra as Peteosthor is in vitro effective against human tubercle bacilli only in very high concentrations (2). About this and the wrong hypothesis of Dr. Troch I reported first in winter 1949 in the medical society of the university of Göttingen, later in the first post-war congress of the German Orthopedic Society in September 1950 in Hannover (1). Here it was first shown with some autoradiographs - 3 were printed in the congress report - that ^{224}Ra is deposited in the growing bone, the normally growing zones of the meta- and epiphyses as into the bone fracture, where it prevents a normal bone structure. I finished my talk with the warning words of a pediatrician against using ^{224}Ra in adolexcence.

Some months later we repeated our warnings at the National Congress of Surgery in the spring of 1951 in München and in the same year experimental data were published (3) and in the following year a critical report on the Thorium-X and peteosthor-therapy (4).

The accumulation of ^{224}Ra in growing bone was for me the reason to prepare the follow-up of the patients. We recorded the medical details, the ^{224}Ra injections and the laboratory data of the patients and took copies for our files.

I left Hildesheim in the autumn of 1949 and paid afterwards some visits to the patients and the staff. The first follow-up we started in 1952 supported by Dr. Bischofsberger, the successor of Dr. Troch as chief of the hospital. We collected all the data available of Peteosthor treated patients, which I could not get as long as Dr. Troch was there in charge. In 1954/55 we traced the patients who had been injected with ^{224}Ra in 1948 and 1949 as children. Visiting the families we tried to clarify the causes of illness or death. In this first follow-up we found the growth retardation as we had already predicted after our animal experiments (Spiess 1951).

Frightening however, was the figure of malignant tumors, which development 4 to 7 years after starting irradiation we described literally the paper published in 1956 'Schwere Strahlenschäden nach der Peteosthorbehandlung von Kindern' (5). Here we published 11 cases of bone sarcoma as late effects of the ^{224}Ra injections.

On benign bone tumors - the exostosis or solitary and multiple osteochondroma as ^{224}Ra late effects - we reported in 1957 (6).

Abroad, I reported in 1956 at the International Congress of Pediatrics in Copenhagen about growth retardation and tumor induction by ^{224}Ra (7). I did the same in 1964 in Brussels in a scientific meeting of EURATOM and in a committee of the British Medical Research Council in London by invitation of Dr. Robin Mole. At the same time Charles Mays had read my paper about Thorium-X induced bone sarcoma and invited me in 1967 his symposium on delayed effects on bone seeking nuclides in Syn Valley/Idaho (8). Afterwards I had repeatedly the pleasure to have him as a guest and coworker here in München. We reported in the International Congress 1970 in Houston and in the last symposion on ^{224}Ra and ^{226}Ra held in Alta, Utah 2 year ago (9).

Now let me discuss our last survey as of August 1976 (Table I): We followed 899 persons with exact information, which were treated with ^{224}Ra: 218 received the ^{224}Ra injections from age 1 to 20 years, 681 as adults. The following diseases are in my opinion late effects of the ^{224}Ra irradia-

TABLE I

FOLLOW-UP OF PATIENTS TREATED WITH ^{224}RA

Total of 1809: no present address: 241; doctor's report without name: 654; examination refused: 16; exact information available: 898 (VIII 76)

	AGE AT TIME OF FIRST TREATMENT 1-20 years	21 years and over	NUMBER total
Number providing information	218	681	899
Report by family doctor or by questionnaire	49	325	374
Personally or hospital examination	107	108	215
Deaths	73	291	364
Causes of death			
Basic disease	11	42	53
Not related to basic disease or malignancy	13	124	173
Unknown	5	29	34
Osteosarcoma	30 (+2L)	16 (+2L)	46 (+4L)
Chondrosarcoma	4	0	4
Other malignancy tumors (Ca)	5 (+1L)	29 (+12L)	34 (+13)
Liver disease	1	17	18
Renal disease	3	31	34
Panmyelophthisis, anaemia	1	2	3
Leukaemia	0	3	3
Other abnormalities			
Benign bone tumors			
Exostoses solitary	7	0	7
Exostoses multiple	20	0	20
Osteochondroblastoma	1	0	1
Osteofibroma	1	0	1
Teeth breaking off	19	11	30
Growth retardation (12 years)	50	0	50
Cataract	11	22	33

ation. They are the isteosarcoma and osteochondrosarcoma, the solitary and multiple exostoses, the growth retardation, the teeth breaking off and most of the cataracts as late effect of the Peteosthor treatment.

Before I discuss the late effects, some remarks as to the soft tissue effects. First to the *kidney* diseases.

About the acute involvement of the kidney of animals or patients injected with ^{224}Ra, I reported in my first papers 1951. In our rabbit experiments as well as in the patients we found frequently after around 15 injections of ^{224}Ra a pathologic urine status with leucocytes, erythrocytes and - as we called them - toxic cylinders. Symptoms of this radiation nephritis we found in 83% of the injected children. They disappeared after reducing the radiation dose. As causes of death we found the more kidney diseases the higher the ^{224}Ra dosage. In our Alta-paper we reported with Chuck Mays among the living and dead men kidney diseases in 3.7% of those injected at lower dosage (below 14.3 μCi ^{224}Ra/kg) and in 4.5% at higher dosage. In women the corresponding incidences were 4.1% and 10.7%.

Although we have some successes, we are reluctant, at this time, to attempt to quantify a dose-response relationship for the ^{224}Ra induction of kidney diseases based on the present data, although the existence of such a relationship seems probable.

If we had time and money it would seem highly desirable to evaluate the kidney and liver function of all living patients by clinical tests.

Concerning the *liver* diseases in our patients we are still more uncertain. No doubt that the enhanced excretion of Urobilinogen in the urine of 29% of our patients - mostly after the 15th injection of ^{224}Ra as Peteosthor - is suggestive for a radiation-induced hepatopathy, but during their treatment, hepatitis was endemic in this hospital. I got it for example also with two relapses because I refused bed rest at this time.

The tendency of the incidence of chronic liver disease to increase with ^{224}Ra dosage suggests that some of the later liver diseases might have been radiation-induced.

In contrast, the incidence of the *soft tissue tumors* is not strikingly higher than the statistically expected figure. Only qualitatively striking is the relatively higher incidence of breast cancers in women and the three times higher incidence than expected for hypernephroma (3 observed/ 1 expected).

The high figure of *cataracts* is striking undoubtedly, especially at an early age, when normally an acquired cataract is extremely rare. Thus, it seems probable that most of the cataracts seen in the 218 patients injected as juveniles and some in the adult patients were induced by the treatment.

As late effects of the previous ^{224}Ra *treatment* it seems likely that all or nearly all of the osteosarcoma and chondrosarcoma, the solitary and multiple exostoses, the osteochondroblastoma, the teeth breaking off and the observed growth retardation are radiation-induced.

REFERENCES

1. Spiess, H., Verhandlungsbericht der Deutschen Orthopädischen Gesellschaft 38. Kongress Hannover 14.-16. September 1950, 205-206.
2. Spiess, H. und C.J. Tietz, Über die Hemmwirkung des Peteosthor und seiner Komponenten auf das Wachstum humaner Tuberkelbakterien in vitro. Klin.Wschr. 28, 420-421 (1950).
3. Spiess, H., Tierexperimentelle Untersuchungen zur parenteralen Thorium-X-Anwendung. Z.exper.Med. 117, 567-586, (1951).
4. Spiess, H., Über Anwendung und Wirkung des Peteosthor bei pulmonaler und extrapulmonaler Tuberkulose im Kindesalter. Zugleich eine allgemeine Stellungnahme zur Thorium-X- und Peteosthor-Therapie. Z. Kinderhk. 70, 213-252 (1952).
5. Spiess, H., Schwere Strahlenschäden nach der Peteosthorbehandlung von Kindern. Dtsch.med.Wschr. 81, 1053-1054 (1956).
6. Spiess, H., Exostotische Dysplasie durch Strahlenwirkung? Dtsch.med.Wschr. 82, 1483-1484 (1957).
7. Spiess, H., Wachstumsstörungen und Geschwülste bei Kindern

durch Strahlen. Proceed. International Congress of Pediatrics, Abstr. No 167, Copenhagen 1956.

8. Spiess, H., ^{224}Ra-induced tumors in children and adults in delayed effects of bone-seeking radionuclides. University of Utah Press, 227-247 (1969).

9. Spiess, H. and C.W. Mays, Bone cancers induced by ^{224}Ra in children and adults, Health Physics (Pergamon Press) 19, 713-729 (1970).

10. Troch, P., Neue Wege des Heilens. Vieweg, Braunschweig, (1949).

Osteogenic sarcomas in mice after ^{224}Ra or ^{226}Ra administrations

Dvorak V.*, V. Kofránek, I. Malátová, D. Bubeníková, V. Klener, V. Svoboda

*Medical Faculty of Hygiene, Charles University; Institute of Hygiene and Epidemiology, Centre of Radiation Hygiene, Prague, Czechoslovakia

SUMMARY

The results of an experiment in which a time distribution of the mean skeletal dose was achieved by repeated ^{224}Ra administrations that was comparable with its time course after a single ^{226}Ra injection are reported.

Ten weeks old SPF female mice were used. The levels administered (μCi/kg): ^{226}Ra - 8.8, 24.6, 70.5; ^{224}Ra - 17.2, 50.5, 167.6, the respective total activities being administered in 150 injections, two injections a week. Numbers of animals: 100 mice in each of the six radium groups, 200 mice served as untreated controls, 200 mice received repeatedly nonactive solution. The course of the mean skeletal dose in the 8.8 μCi/kg ^{226}Ra group did not deviate from the region delineated by the courses of dose levels in two ^{224}Ra groups (50.5 μCi/kg, 167.6 μCi/kg). Osteogenic sarcomas occurrence ^{226}Ra group: 19%; ^{224}Ra groups: 80%, 56%.

The experimental set-up enabled a direct comparison of osteogenic sarcoma occurrence in mice under conditions of comparable time course of the mean skeletal dose from repeated ^{224}Ra or single ^{226}Ra injections; ^{224}Ra was found to be three to four times more efficient than ^{226}Ra in the region of comparable doses. The evaluation of the role of the differences in soft tissue exposures is still in progress.

INTRODUCTION

A long-term program of studies on the time and space distribution of the dose from ^{224}Ra and ^{226}Ra in relation to delayed effects was launched at the Centre of Radiation Hygiene, Prague, several years ago. The ^{224}Ra section of this program has centred on the kinetics of radium and its daughter products and the induction of osteogenic sarcomas in mice after repeated administrations of ^{224}Ra.

The results of an experiment in which a time distribution of the mean skeletal dose was achieved by repeated ^{224}Ra administrations that was comparable with its time distribution after a single ^{226}Ra injection are reported in this paper. These results will be related to the results of a parallel ^{226}Ra study. The experimental set-up is schematically shown in Table I.

TABLE I

THE ACTIVITIES OF ^{226}RA AND OF ^{224}RA ADMINISTERED

N - numbers of animals per groups
TA, TB, TC - the levels of ^{224}Ra
UD, UE, UF - the levels of ^{226}Ra
UK - untreated controls
TK - non-active solution repeatedly injected

^{226}Ra N	^{226}Ra μCi/kg	Group	^{224}Ra μCi/kg	^{224}Ra N
		TA	17.2	100
100	8.8	UD — TB	50.5	100
100	24.6	UE — TC	167.6	100
100	70.5	UF		
200	—	UK TK	—	200

This communication is confined to the occurrence of osteogenic sarcomas; a more detailed evaluation of the other biological parameters related to the relative radiotoxicity of the radium isotopes will be presented in the paper by Kofránek et al. (2).

MATERIAL AND METHODS

Ten weeks old SPF female mice of Czechoslovak provenance, strain ICR (Swiss), were used. Radium isotopes in ionic form were injected in 0.1 ml volumes of solution, pH 3-4, with $CaCl_2$ as a carrier.

^{224}Ra was obtained from ^{228}Th (Amersham Laboratories) in a generator-type device (5). A total of 150 injections were given per animal, two injections a week, the activities being administered in three levels, each to a group of 100 mice. The total activities given are presented in Table I, a more detailed information of activities given is expressed in Table II and Figure 1.

TABLE II

THE INDIVIDUAL ACTIVITIES OF ^{224}RA INJECTED (ABRIDGED)

Injection No.	Time from the 1st inj. (days)	Activity of ^{224}Ra given (μCi per animal) TA	TB	TC
1	0	18.40	48.65	130.5
2	4	15.70	41.00	131.30
3	7	15.70	43.00	142.20
4	11	15.85	48.85	135.55
5	14	16.10	44.75	144.90
10	32	9.50	25.50	76.65
20	67	5.95	17.05	53.90
50*	172	9.75	12.00	80.90

* Constant values were administered in injections No. 51 to 150; the alternate planned values in the TB level were 10.9 μCi per animal (4-day interval) and 8.1 μCi per animal (3-day interval).

^{226}Ra (Soviet provenance) was administered in three fractions within one week, also in three levels of activity given to groups of 100 animals each. These activities are presented in Table I.

Two hundred mice served as untreated controls, 200 animals received non-active solution. Parameters followed were activ-

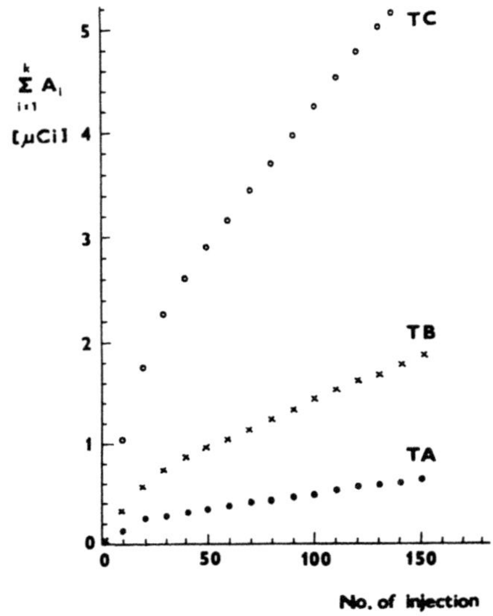

FIGURE 1

Cumulative activities of ^{224}Ra administered in levels TA, TB, TC

ity of administered solutions, gamma spectrometric measurements in vivo, contamination of administered solutions with ^{228}Th, health condition, death rate, weight, hematological findings, autopsy, X-ray findings on the skeleton, and histology. Mice of all groups were followed up until death.

RESULTS AND DISCUSSION

Figure 2 presents the mean skeletal doses for the individual groups of ^{224}Ra mice in relation to the doses for mice contaminated with ^{226}Ra, and Figure 3 presents the mean skeletal doses after single administration of ^{224}Ra for mice of different age. The doses were calculated according to the formula

$$D(t) = \sum_{j=1} E_j \sum_{i=1}^{n} A_i \int_{t_i}^{t} \frac{f_j(\tau - t_i)}{m(\tau)} d\tau$$

where

i	is the number of administrations
j	is index of radionuclide contributing to dose
t_i	time of i-th administration
$m(\tau)$	weight of mouse skeleton
$f_j(\tau)$	relative retention function of j-th radionuclide
E_j	energy of alpha particles
A_i	activity given at i-th administration

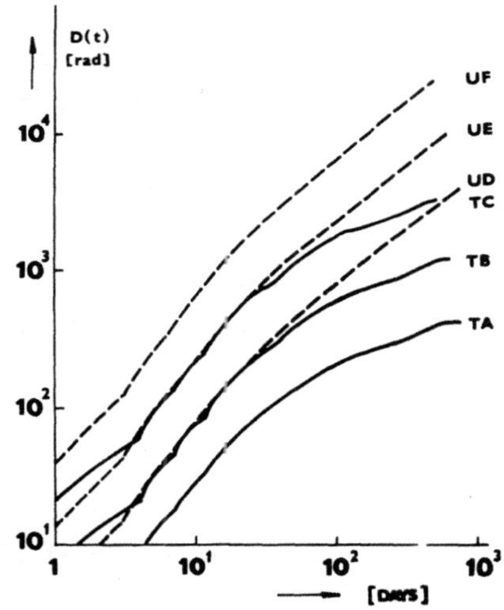

FIGURE 2

Time-course of the mean skeletal doses after repeated injections of ^{224}Ra (TA, TB, TC) or single injections of ^{226}Ra (UD, UE, UF)

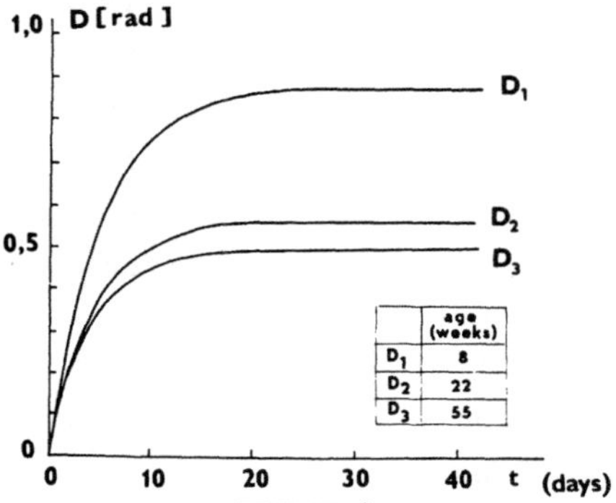

FIGURE 3

Time-course of mean skeletal doses after single injection of 1 μCi of ^{224}Ra in mice of different age

The mean skeletal dose from radium isotopes and their daughter products was calculated on the following assumptions: only the energy of alpha particles was considered (energy of beta-particles and recoil nuclei was neglected); all the energy of alpha-particles originated in the skeleton is absorbed in the skeleton.

The experimentally determined relations of kinetic parameters to age and previous exposure were allowed for in the calculations (3).

The level of ^{224}Ra corresponding to the highest level of the ^{226}Ra burden was not administered because in a previous experiment in which ^{224}Ra had been given 40 times in injections of 0.2 μCi per mouse, with the mean skeletal dose lying on the level of UF dose, the group of 75 mice died out within 11 months showing symptoms of subacute radiation damage and no osteogenic sarcomas were proved. Relatively high levels of ^{224}Ra activities were chosen in order to achieve dose values at which a high induction of osteosarcomas could be expected.

The target of our ^{224}Ra program was to achieve, by multiple administrations of the isotope, the required course of the mean skeletal dose from ^{224}Ra and its daughter products and reach levels suitable for osteosarcomas studies. In view of the demands on time and capacity involved, a threestage approach was adopted, as follows:

1. To determine by single injection experiments retention data in relatively young mice and to carry out a pilot experiment with repeated administrations.
2. To obtain, in a long-term experiment, further dosimetric information for the formation of a more realistic administration schema, and to evaluate delayed effects, particularly occurrence of osteogenic sarcomas, as related to the results of a parallel study with ^{226}Ra.
3. To apply the injection schedule derived at stage 2 in other long-term studies.

In our opinion, already the administration schema used at stage 2 permitted to regard as comparable the course of skeletal doses in groups TC and TB, and in group UD which had been given ^{226}Ra (Figure 2). Simultaneously, data were obtained for the formulation of a more exact administration schema (4).

Contaminants of the solutions injected, especially ^{228}Th from which ^{224}Ra is separated, may also contribute to the skeletal dose. ^{228}Th was measured in samples from each separation carried out. The values determined, expressed as radiochemical impurity, amounted to 10^{-2} to 10^{-3} per cent of ^{224}Ra activities. Preliminary results of a long-term complementary experiment with repeated administrations of ^{228}Th in three levels indicate that its contribution to the skeletal dose in the experiment reported has no significant effect on the induction of osteogenic sarcomas in the ^{224}Ra animals.

The occurrence of osteogenic sarcomas in the individual groups is presented in Tables III and IV.

A complex evaluation of the autopsy, X-ray and histological findings in individual mice served as the criterion for considering a tumour to be osteosarcoma. In doubtful cases the decision was based upon histology. Presumably, a high detection rate was achieved using the combination of the methods. Detection could further be enhanced using serial sections of all bones, evidence for which can also be furnished in our material by sporadic findings of spinal osteosarcomas diagnosed at histological examination of spinal cords and backbones removed to determine the cause of paresis of the distal limbs. These sarcomas were not apparent either at autopsy or at the X-ray reading. Owing to its extreme demands on time and capacity, this method was not used in the present study.

Among 400 non-active mice, one osteogenic sarcoma was found.

Since the course of the mean skeletal dose in group UD did not diverge from the band delimited by the course of dose levels in TB and TC, the dose within this area can be regarded as comparable. Single injections of ^{224}Ra lead to the development of osteogenic sarcomas (1), with the considerable fraction of dose being delivered during the

TABLE III

Occurrence of osteogenic sarcomas in ^{224}Ra mice

Weeks after 1st administr.	TA			TB			TC		
	N †	N mice with o.s.	N o.s.	N †	N mice with o.s.	N o.s.	N †	N mice with o.s.	N o.s.
4	-	-	-	-	-	-	-	-	-
8	1	-	-	-	-	-	-	-	-
12	-	-	-	-	-	-	1	-	-
16	-	-	-	2	-	-	3	-	-
20	1	-	-	2	-	-	2	-	-
24	3	-	-	4	1	1	5	-	-
28	3	-	-	2	-	-	5	-	-
32	8	-	-	9	1	1	7	1	-
36	2	-	-	7	3	3	6	4	4
40	4	-	-	6	2	2	11	6	7
44	8	1	1	13	8	9	12	6	8
48	3	-	-	4	1	1	12	6	7
52	6	2	2	9	6	7	8	3	3
56	5	2	2	14	9	15	13	10	15
60	7	1	1	11	7	10	9	5	6
64	7	-	-	6	5	12	4	2	4
68	5	1	1	4	3	5	1	1	2
72	6	2	2	3	3	5	1	-	-
76	5	1	1	1	-	-	-	-	-
80	8	4	4	2	2	9	-	-	-
84	6	2	4	-	-	-	-	-	-
88	2	-	-	1	-	-	-	-	-
92	5	3	3	-	-	-	-	-	-
96	2	1	1	-	-	-	-	-	-
100	-	-	-	-	-	-	-	-	-
104	2	1	1	-	-	-	-	-	-
Σ	100	21	23	100	51	80	100	43	56

N † - Number of mice died or killed   o.s. - osteogenic sarcoma

TABLE IV

Occurrence of osteogenic sarcomas in ^{226}Ra mice

Weeks after 1st administr.	TA			TB			TC		
	N †	N mice with o.s.	N o.s.	N †	N mice with o.s.	N o.s.	N †	N mice with o.s.	N o.s.
4	-	-	-	-	-	-	-	-	-
8	2	-	-	1	-	-	2	-	-
12	-	-	-	-	-	-	-	-	-
16	1	-	-	1	-	-	-	-	-
20	2	-	-	4	-	-	2	-	-
24	2	-	-	4	-	-	7	-	-
28	4	-	-	4	-	-	7	-	-
32	2	-	-	5	-	-	13	-	-
36	2	-	-	2	1	1	14	-	-
40	4	-	-	3	1	1	8	1	1
44	5	-	-	6	3	3	22	1	1
48	5	1	1	11	6	8	11	3	3
52	5	-	-	6	2	2	4	2	2
56	4	1	1	9	4	7	8	-	-
60	11	4	4	8	3	7	1	-	-
64	14	7	7	8	5	5	-	-	-
68	14	1	1	14	9	12	1	-	-
72	6	1	1	4	1	1	-	-	-
76	5	1	1	4	3	3	-	-	-
80	4	-	-	5	2	2	-	-	-
84	3	1	2	1	-	-	-	-	-
88	2	-	-	-	-	-	-	-	-
92	1	1	1	-	-	-	-	-	-
96	1	-	-	-	-	-	-	-	-
100	-	-	-	-	-	-	-	-	-
104	1	-	-	-	-	-	-	-	-
Σ	100	18	19	100	40	52	100	7	7

N † - Number of mice died or killed   o.s. - osteogenic sarcoma

first 2 weeks following administration. Hence it may be assumed that in our conditions, where the levels of activities administered at the beginning of the experiment were approximately one order higher than in the last injections, the activities administered in the first days and decades of days contributed considerably to the total yield of the osteogenic sarcomas induced. During this initial period up to approximately the 30th day the course of dose in the UD group did not differ by more than 10% from the course in TB, and also up to 100th day the increase of the UD values as compared to TB was rather slow (Fig. 2).

Direct comparison under conditions of comparable skeletal dose showed that ^{224}Ra is three to four times more effective in osteogenic sarcoma induction than ^{226}Ra. In view of the time courses of doses it is more reasonable rather to consider the higher value.

Moreover, the different exposure of the soft tissues which results from the repeated administration of ^{224}Ra in comparison to a triplex injection of ^{226}Ra may change the yield of osteosarcomas in mice exposed to ^{224}Ra more than in mice given ^{226}Ra. Evaluation of survival curves and of other parameters of biological response is consistent in that groups with a higher level of exposure display more pronounced consequences for the basic functions of the organism. The differences between individual levels of administered activities of the same isotope and also between mouse groups receiving different radium isotopes are obviously reflected in the actually observed numbers of osteosarcomas in the individual groups. An evaluation in greater detail of the differences in the biological parameters studied and their relation to damages whose occurrence is of a stochastic nature will be given in the paper by Kofránek et al. (2).

The experimental set-up enabled a direct comparison of osteogenic sarcoma occurrence after ^{224}Ra and ^{226}Ra administrations to an identical material; ^{224}Ra was found to be 3-4 times more efficient than ^{226}Ra in the region of comparable doses. The evaluation of the role of the differences in soft tissue exposures is still in progress.

REFERENCES

1. Hug, O., W. Gössner, W.A. Müller, A. Luz, B. Hinderinger, Production of osteosarcomas in mice and rats by incorporation of radium-224. Proc.Symp.on Radiation-Induced Cancer, p. 393-409, Athens 1969.
2. Kofránek, V., V. Dvořák, V. Klener, A. Sedlák, V. Svoboda, D. Bubeníková, Z. Onyskowová, J. Thomas, V. Lenger, J. Salava, Biological effects of ^{224}Ra and ^{226}Ra and their relative radiotoxicity in mice. Proc.Sympt. on 'Biological Effects of ^{224}Ra', Neuherberg 1976.
3. Malátová, I., V. Dvořák, Retention of ^{224}Ra and ^{212}Pb in skeletons of mice. Proc.4th Conf.Radiat.Hyg., Jasná, p. 217-227, Purkyně Med.Res.Postgrad.Press, Hr.Králové 1971.
4. Malátová, I., J. Thomas, Opredělenije dozy v skeletě myši posle razovovo i povtornovo vveděniia radioizotopov radija. Sbornik I. Radiobiologičeskoj konferencii socialističeskich stran, Bedřichov, 1974 - in press.
5. Rajtora, J., I. Malátová, A rapid milking method for the preparation of ^{224}Ra from ^{228}Th solution. Radiochem.Radioanal.Letters 6, 227-236 (1971).

Biological effects of ^{224}Ra and ^{226}Ra and their relative radiotoxicity in mice

Kofránek V., V. Dvořák*, V. Klener, A. Sedlák, V. Svoboda, D. Bubeníková, Z. Onyskowová, J. Thomas, V. Lenger, J. Salava
Institute of Hygiene and Epidemiology, Centre of Radiation Hygiene;
* Medical Faculty of Hygiene, Charles University, Prague, Czechoslovakia

SUMMARY

Groups of ten-week-old ICR SPF female mice were treated intraperitoneally with 3 levels of ^{224}Ra and ^{226}Ra activities. The administration scheme provided the skeletal dose from ^{224}Ra and its daughter products (T series of mice) comparable to that resulting from a single injection of ^{226}Ra (U series of mice). Three hundred mice in each experimental series and 400 controls, kept under standard conditions till their death, were evaluated. The mean survival time of mice was found to become shorter in dependent on the increasing quantity of administered radionuclides and in mice with comparable skeletal doses some biological effects of ^{224}Ra were found to surpass those of ^{226}Ra. All mice were examined roentgenographically and histopathologically after their death. Osteosarcoma induction was observed more frequently after injections of ^{224}Ra than after ^{226}Ra incorporation. Only a single bone tumour was detected in the group of control mice.

The presented experimental findings seem to lead to a general conclusion that, at the same skeletal dose, the relative radiotoxicity of ^{224}Ra is about 4 times higher than the toxicity of ^{226}Ra. The possibility of how to compare experimental results obtained in various laboratories is also discussed.

INTRODUCTION

As a part of our radiation research programme carried out to study the relationship of temporal and spatial distribution of skeletal doses to the late biological effects of radionuclides, we have conducted a comparative study in mice using two radium isotopes of different half-lives. Long-term *experiments were conducted on mice which received repeatedly injections of* ^{224}*Ra* (T series of mice) *with the objective to achieve a time course of the skeletal dose comparable to the time course after a single administration of* ^{226}*Ra* (U series of mice). The levels of administered activities, their administration scheme, the course of skeletal doses as well as the rate of osteosarcoma production are presented in a paper by Dvořák et al. (2).

MATERIAL AND METHODS

Ten-weeks-old ICR SPF female mice of Czechoslovak provenance were divided into 6 experimental groups (each consisting of 100 animals) and into 2 control groups (each with 200 mice). 300 Mice received repeated doses of ^{224}Ra, 300 experimental mice were given ^{226}Ra, 200 mice were repeatedly injected with non-active solution (TK group of mice) and 200 control animals remained untreated (UK group of mice). The isotope of ^{224}Ra, repeatedly obtained from ^{228}Th, as well as ^{226}Ra were administered intraperitoneally in the form of chlorides at pH 3-4, carrier $CaCl_2$, in three levels of activity within the range of one order.

^{224}Ra was administered in 150 injections at a rate of 2 injections per week, ^{226}Ra was given in three fractions within 1 week, the respective doses for ^{224}Ra being 17.2, 50.5 and 167.6 μCi/kg and for ^{226}Ra 8.8, 24.6 and 70.5 μCi/kg b.w. All the animals involved in this experiment were kept under standard conditions (6) and observed until their extinction.

The following biological criteria were evaluated: health status, mortality rate, body weight, peripheral blood changes (using routine hematological techniques), roentgenography of the skeleton and histopathology of body organs and tumours.

RESULTS

The numbers of mice, gradually decreasing by dead or 'ante finem' sacrificed animals, are given in Figure 1. In contrast to the control animals (TK and UK), the experimental groups of mice with incorporated radium isotopes exhibited steeper

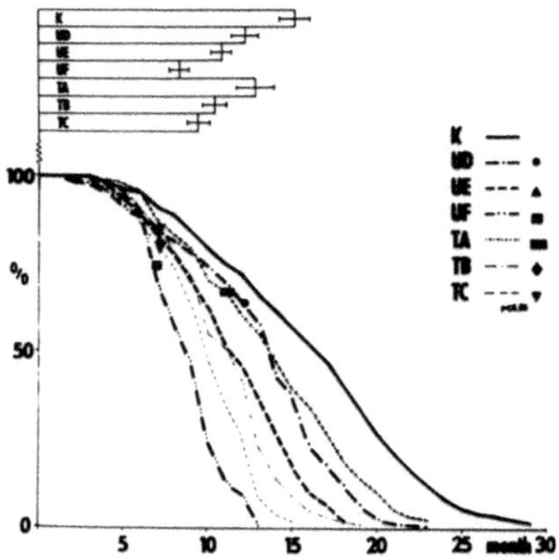

FIGURE 1

Survival curves in groups of mice with incorporated ^{224}Ra (T-series) and ^{226}Ra (U-series), indicating the mean survival time and the period when the values started to be statistically different from those in control ($p < 0.05$)
Dose comparable groups of mice: TD = UD, TC = UE

survival curves dependent on the level of administered activities. In groups of mice with comparable ^{224}Ra and ^{226}Ra skeletal doses (TB = UD and TC = UE) the survival curves appeared to be steeper in mice with incorporated ^{224}Ra than in those that had received ^{226}Ra, which is also demonstrated in the table with mean survival time values for individual animal groups (in days):

TK	UK	TA	TB	TC	UD	UE	UF
446.6	458.1	382.6	312.2	283.1	365.2	324.5	249.2

The body weight values in experimental mice (Fig. 2) deviated during the experiment from the weight values of the control animals, which was particularly evident from the 2nd month after the first radionuclide administration in groups of mice with the highest activity levels. It is also apparent that besides the dependence on increasing levels of administered radionuclide activities there was also an apparent dependence on the type of administered isotope.

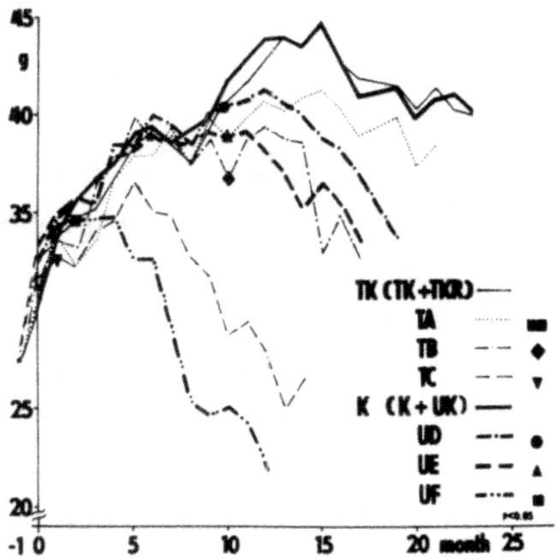

FIGURE 2

Body weight curves in groups of mice with incorporated ^{224}Ra (T-series) and ^{226}Ra (U-series), indicating the period when the values started to be statistically different from those in the controls ($p < 0.05$)
Dose comparable groups of mice: TB = UD, TC = UE

In groups of mice with comparable skeletal doses there were found lower weight values in mice with ^{224}Ra than in those incorporated with ^{226}Ra.

Histopathological examination of 400 control mice revealed only a single case of spontaneous osteosarcoma (Table I).

TABLE I

OCCURRENCE OF HISTOPATHOLOGICAL CHANGES IN THE CONTROLS (TK AND UK) AND IN MICE OF THE SERIES T (^{224}RA) AND U (^{226}RA)

Findings	N	TK 200 %	UK 200 %	TA 100 %	TB 100 %	TC 100 %	UD 100 %	UE 100 %	UF 100 %
Malignant tumours:									
Osteosarcomas		-	0.5	23	80	56	19	52	7
(Mice with osteosarcomas)		-	0.5	21	51	43	18	40	7
Hemoblastoses		36	26	25	22	23	19	27	22
Carcinomas		24	31.5	27	16	9	35	20	4
Others		3.5	6.5	7	2	4	4	6	4
Benign tumours:									
Lung adenomas		32	34.5	25	30	32	20	37	28
Regressive changes:									
Amyloidosis		42	26.5	44	32	22	22	7	3
Spleen atrophy		-	-	3	2	6	1	2	25
Nephropathy		-	-	-	-	-	-	-	72

On the other hand, there was detected a high incidence rate of other malignancies, especially hemoblastoses. Of solid malignant tumours there was a prevalence of adenocarcinomas localized in the lungs and mammary glands. Benign tumours were usually represented by pulmonary adenomas, regressive changes were mostly characterized by the occurrence of amyloidosis.

The mice exposed to radium isotopes differed significantly from the controls in the occurrence of osteosarcomas - see Figure 3. Parallel occurrence of two or more osteosarcomas in bones of one animal was detectable in mice of both the groups (T and U), in mice with incorporated ^{224}Ra being always more frequent. This occurrence of multifocal osteogenic sarcomas was not observed in mice of the group UF. Excluding osteosarcomas and hemoblastoses, the total number of other malignant tumours was found to decline in individual groups of mice in dependence on increasing levels of incorporated ^{224}Ra and ^{226}Ra activities. In mice with the highest activity of ^{226}Ra (group UF) there were observed qualitative-

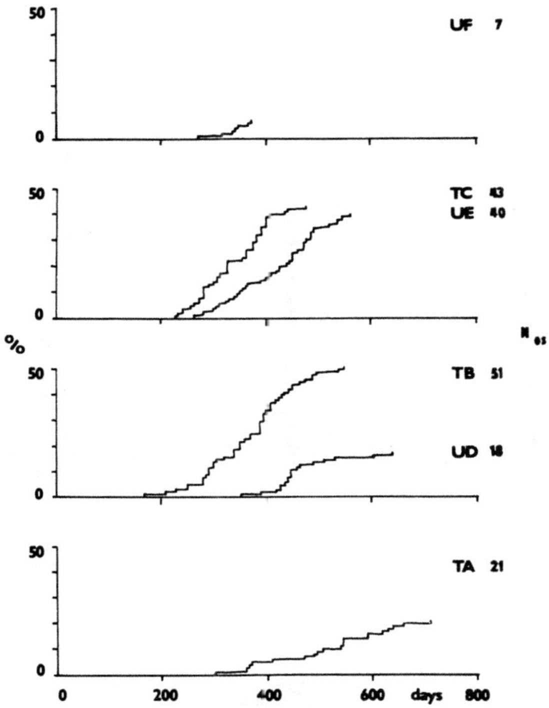

FIGURE 3

Cumulative incidence of osteosarcomas in mice after repeated injections of ^{224}Ra (T-series) and single injection of ^{226}Ra (U-series). Each experimental group of mice consists of 100 experimental animals. Dose comparable groups of mice: TB = UD, TC = UE
% - percentage of mice with osteosarcoma

ly different changes, as for example heavy regressive changes of the spleen and kidneys. The spectrum of other pathological changes remained about the same in experimental and control animals, excepting a higher incidence rate of amyloidosis observed in mice of the group T, however, the number of amyloid-bearing mice was found to decline with the increasing radiation levels.

Parallel experiments with ^{224}Ra and ^{226}Ra incorporation revealed also some differences in the localization of osteogenic sarcomas in mice with comparable skeletal doses. Figures 4a and 4b show schematically that the frequency rate

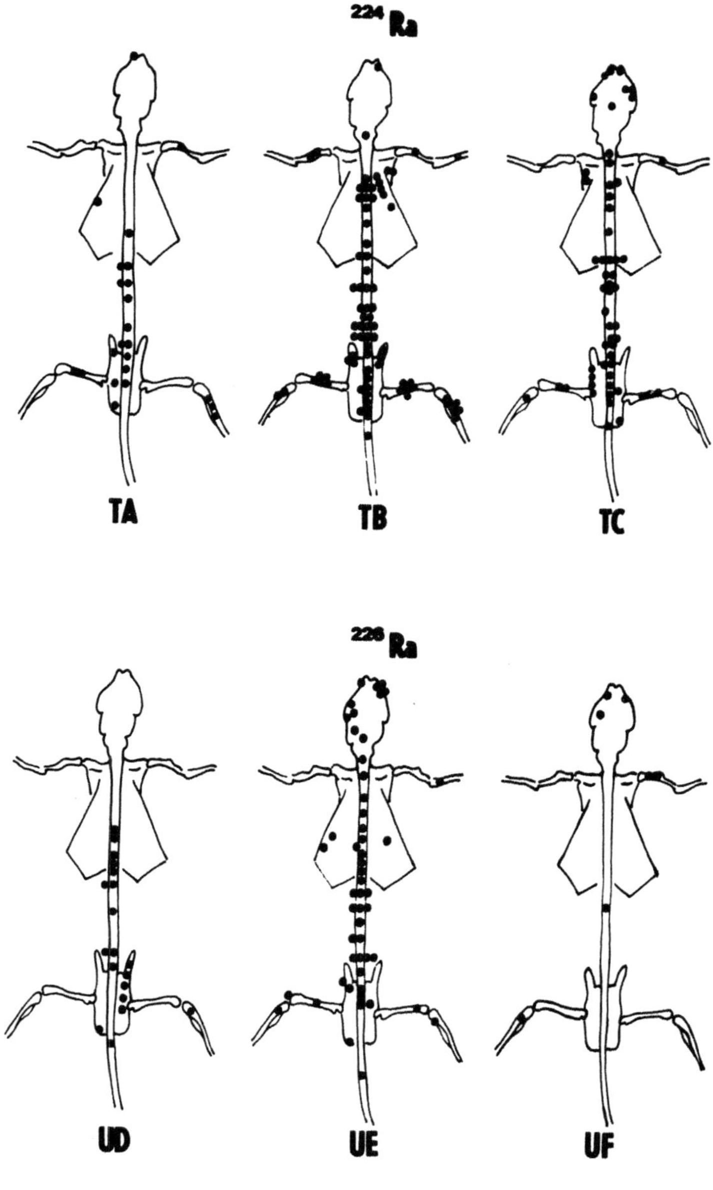

FIGURE 4a, 4b

Anatomic localization of skeletal osteosarcoma in mice of the series T (^{224}Ra) and series U (^{226}Ra) Dose comparable groups of mice: TB = UD, TC = UE

of vertebral and pelvic tumours remained practically on the same level of statistical significance (66.7% and 64.1%). However, in the bones of limbs and skull there occurred significant percentual differences in osteosarcoma distribution: in mice with incorporated ^{224}Ra there was a higher prevalence of limb (especially hind limb) tumours (22.7% against 11.6% after ^{226}Ra) and, on the contrary, a lower frequency rate of skull osteosarcomas (6.3% against 16.6% after ^{226}Ra) localized mainly in jaw-bones, particularly in the mandible. The only exception was the group of the mice with the highest level of administered ^{224}Ra in which maxilla osteosarcomas prevailed.

Our experimental conditions enabled us to compare, on the basis of skeletal dose comparability, the relative radiotoxicity after a single dose of ^{226}Ra and after repeated injections of ^{224}Ra. Of several methods available for the calculation of relative radiotoxicity values we decided to determine the ratio of initial percentage of the mice with osteosarcomas (M) to the relative levels of selected radionuclide activities (D_{rel}), as indicated in Figure 5. From this ratio of initial slopes it may be derived that the value of relative radiotoxicity of ^{224}Ra in regard to ^{226}Ra is about 3-5.

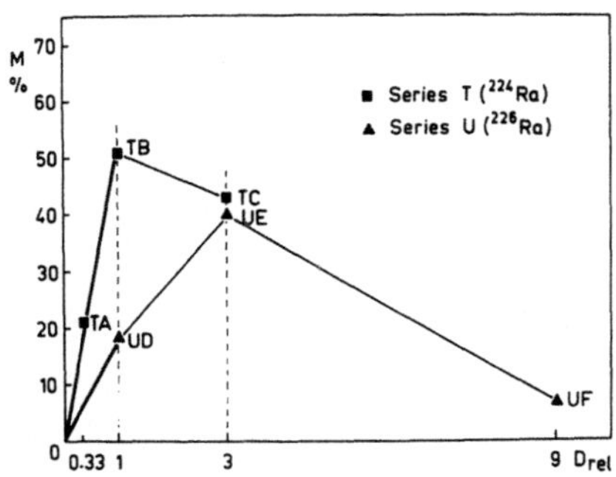

FIGURE 5

Percentage of mice with osteosarcomas in dependent in relative dose levels (D_{rel}). The ratio of initial slopes (thick) is of the value of 3-5 (radiotoxicity of ^{224}Ra relative to ^{226}Ra). In groups of mice TC and UF there is a decreasing tendency to osteosracoma production: therefore they are not included to the relative radiotoxicity calculations.

DISCUSSION

Comparability of skeletal doses in ^{224}Ra and ^{226}Ra parallel experiments enabled to compare the biological effects of the two radium isotopes and to determine their relative radiotoxicity.

As indicated in Figure 1, the course of survival time curves does not seem to imply the presence of microbial infections in mice, which was also proved by randomly conducted bacteriological examinations. The body weights of experimental animals (Figure 2) tended to deviate from the control values, which was quite apparent starting the 2nd month after the beginning of experiment in groups of the mice with the highest levels of radium activities. Presented data indicate a dependence of these changes on increasing levels of incorporated activities. In mice with comparable skeletal doses a more severe response was always found in mice with incorporated ^{224}Ra. Life span values and body weight changes may be considered as the complex indicators reflecting the all mechanisms of radiation damage of the basic body functions.

If we analyse the group of mice with the highest level of incorporated ^{226}Ra (UF) we can see that it apparently differs from all other groups and in all the studied parameters, showing a shortest life span (Figure 1), a most pronounced loss of body weight (Figure 2) and gross changes both in white and red blood cells of peripheral blood (13). The analysis of reduced survival time seems rather to indicate that the time distribution of deaths and pathological changes found in this group of mice are characteristic for chronic radiation injury in which supressed blood formation, however significant, is only one of more pathogenetic components. Quite conciderable heavy morphological changes observed in the kidneys and spleen of these mice may be causatively ascribed to radionuclide retention which was extremely high in all the studied organs early after injection of ^{226}Ra.

A high spontaneous incidence of hemoblastoses substantially reduced the possibility to analyse more properly the ability of ^{224}Ra and ^{226}Ra isotopes to induce osteosarcomas. However, in animals with incorporated ^{226}Ra an earlier development of malignancies of the blood-forming system was observed, as has been already reported by Klener et al. (5) in a different mouse strain.

As we can see from the cumulative incidence of osteosarcomas in mice (Figure 3), after repeated injections of ^{224}Ra there is evident a higher as well as an earlier osteosarcoma incidence than in dose comparable groups of mice with incorporated ^{226}Ra.

From Figures 4a and 4b it follows that the two radium isotopes induced osteogenic sarcomas predominantly in axial mouse skeletons, in case of ^{224}Ra in addition also in the bones of limbs. A generally higher incidence rate of ^{224}Ra induced bone tumours (Tabel I) might result from repeated administrations of low radionuclide activities and consequently from the irradiation of newly originated progeny of osteoprogenitor cells in endosteum. In addition to it, there was detected a higher incidence of osteosarcomas in the hind limbs of mice with incorporated ^{224}Ra. It might be of interest in this connection that parallelly conducted experiment with ^{3}H-TDR labelling exhibited a higher turnover rate of osteoprogenitor cells in the endosteal zone of long bones, namely in distal femoral epiphysis (8), where there was also radiochemically detected the highest retention of ^{226}Ra (7).

Due to the fact that the level of ^{226}Ra skeletal dose in UD groups of mice varied in the course of the whole experiment between relatively narrow limits given by the course of ^{224}Ra dose levels in TB and TC groups of mice, it is possible to conclude, on the basis of a direct comparison of osteosarcoma occurrence, that the relative toxicity of ^{224}Ra for the given dose levels is 3-4 times higher than of ^{226}Ra - see the time course of skeletal doses in the communication by Dvořák et al. (2).

Since the mean skeletal doses exhibit somewhat different courses in groups of mice with repeatedly incorporated ^{224}Ra and in those after a single administration of ^{226}Ra, it is important which time interval after the administration is chosen to represent the dose of interest. Figure 5 shows the number of mice with osteosarcomas, related to the relative dose D_{rel} 1:3:9 (as intended in the study), regardless of neither the contributions to the total dose in the late periods of the experiment, nor deviations from the selected activity levels. The lay-out of the relative dose D_{rel} into the diagram was facilitated by the fact that during the period of about 100 days after the first injection there were detected no significant differences in the mean skeletal doses between UD-TB groups of mice (day 100 - approx. 800 rad) and UE-TC groups of mice (day 100 - approx. 2400 rad). Provided that the dose-effect relationship is not curvilinear it is then possible to estimate, from the ratio of initial slopes, the relative toxicity of ^{224}Ra as being 3-5 times higher than of ^{226}Ra.

The problems connected with dose-effect relationship and with the relative toxicity in a long-term experiment have become a subject of concern to quite a number of investigators (1, 4, 9, 11, 12).

For a better comparison of our data with the results reported by Mays et al. (9) we have chosen the dose related to the 140th day prior to the death of experimental mice. In spite of differences in the strains of mice and in their environmental conditions there is (Figure 6) an evident agreement in ^{226}Ra reference values and in an increased occurrence of osteosarcomas after ^{224}Ra incorporation. The value of the coefficient of risk, expressed as the frequency of osteogenic sarcomas per 10^6 mice and per 1 rad of the mean skeletal dose, is in our experimental setting equalled to 70 for ^{226}Ra and to about 600 for ^{224}Ra. Mays et al. (9) reported also the value of 70 for ^{226}Ra. The relative toxicity derived from the ratio of the coefficients of risk (70:600) is in the region of 8-9. If we assume that the accumulated dose of incorporated radionuclides in the later period of mice life is less effective in inducing osteosarcomas, then the lower values of risk coefficients, derived from the direct comparison of data from the TB-TC and UD

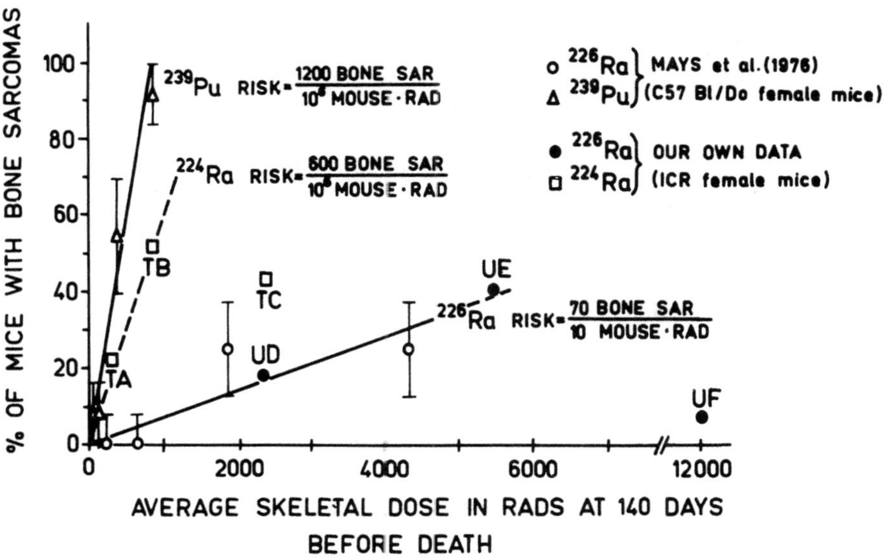

FIGURE 6

Estimated osteosarcoma risk in our experiment with ^{224}Ra and ^{226}Ra compared with findings by Mays - diagram according to Mays et al. (9)

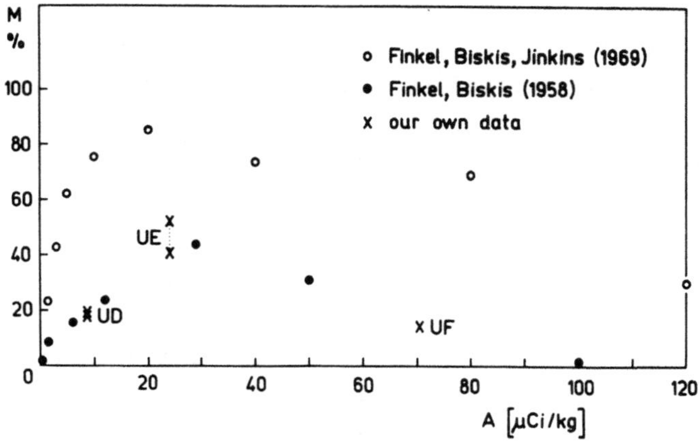

FIGURE 7

Comparison of our experimental induction of osteosarcomas after ^{226}Ra injection (UD, UE and UF groups of mice) with findings by Finkel et al. (3, 4)
Each doubled symbol in UD and UE group of mice represents: Mice with osteosarcomas (lower symbol) and whole number of osteosarcomas (upper symbol)

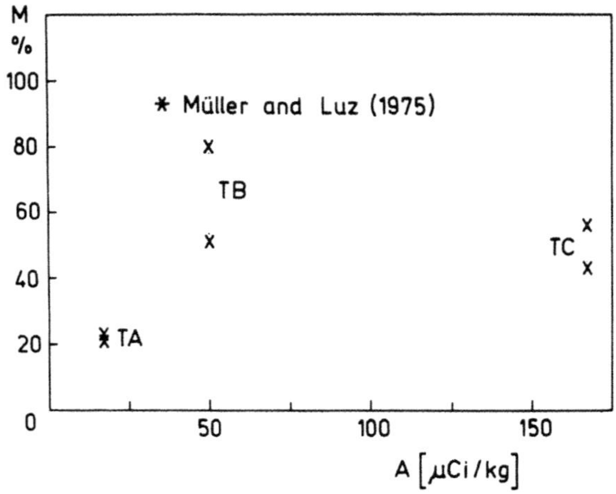

FIGURE 8

Comparison of our experimental induction of osteosarcomas after repeated ^{224}Ra injections (TA, TB and TC groups of mice) with findings by Müller and Luz (10) Each doubled symbol in TA, TB and TC group of mice represents: Mice with osteosarcomas (lower symbol) and whole number of osteosarcomas (upper symbol)

groups of mice and from the initial slopes (Figure 5), seem to be more realistic.

The comparison of our ^{226}Ra data with the results of both experiments reported by Finkel et al. (3, 4), is presented in Figure 7. These results, however, are rather a demonstration of difficulties when comparing data from different laboratories, regardless of coincidental agreement in some parameters.

The only available data which were obtained in experiments with mice given repeated doses of ^{224}Ra (10) are hardly comparable because of different experimental conditions, particularly the age of the animals when starting the ^{224}Ra exposure (4, respectively 10 weeks). The osteosarcoma incidence of authors Müller and Luz (10), who studied long-term effects of repeated ^{224}Ra doses (72 injections within 36 weeks), as well as our results, are given in Figure 8. In spite of the fact that these authors calculate the skeletal dose in a somewhat different way, the resulting mean skeletal doses per unit of incorporated activity were found to be comparable. Nevertheless, it seems that the yields of osteosarcoma production in our experimental conditions were lower than in the Neuherberg laboratory.

ACKNOWLEDGEMENT

This extensive experimental programme has been based on a close cooperation with a team of more than 25 co-workers from the Laboratory of radiotoxicity and Laboratory of gamma-spectrometry.

The authors wish to express their greatest esteem for the help of these unnamed colleagues without whom this demanding research in the field of radium isotopes toxicity could not have been accomplished.

REFERENCES

1. Blair, F.A., Radiation dose-time relations for induction of osteosarcomas in mice and dogs and their bearing on maximal permissible burden of ^{90}Sr in man. Health Phys. 23, 759-769 (1972).
2. Dvořák, V., V. Kofránek, I. Malátová, D. Bubeníková, V. Klener, V. Svoboda, Osteogenic sarcomas in mice after ^{224}Ra or ^{226}Ra administrations. Proc.Symp. on 'Biological Effects of ^{224}Ra', Neuherberg 1976.
3. Finkel, M.P., B.O. Biskis, The induction of malignant bone tumours in mice by radioisotopes. Acta Univ.c. Cancrum 15, 99 (1955).
4. Finkel, M.P., B.O. Biskis, P.B. Jinkins, Toxicity of Ra-226 in mice. Proc.Sympt. on 'Radiation-Induced Cancer, p. 369-391, Vienna 1969.
5. Klener, V., V. Kofránek, Z. Onyskowová, R. Holuša, V. Svoboda, The late effects induced by ^{226}Ra in mice. Proc.Second European IRPA Congress, p. 227-230, Budapest 1972.

6. Kofránek, V., J. Tábořík, Special unit for a long-termed stabling of small laboratory animals with incorporated radionuclides. Zdrav.tech.vzduchotech. 15, 71-74 (1972).
7. Kofránek, V., O. Pařízak, J. Machek, J. Thomas, J. Hanzlík, Distribution of ^{226}Ra in the bones of mice. Acta Radiol. Ther.Phys.Biol. 12, 353-367 (1973).
8. Kofránek V., O. Pařízek, V. Svoboda, D. Bubeníková, J. Machek, ^{3}H-TDR labelling of osteoprogenitor cells after ^{226}Ra incorporation in mice. Acta Radiol.Ther. Phys.Biol. - in press.
9. Mays, C.W., H. Spiess, G.N. Taylor, R.D. Lloyd, W.S.S. Jee, S.S. McFarland, D.H. Taysum, T.W. Brammer, D. Brammer, T.A. Pollard, Estimated risk to human bone from ^{239}Pu. In: Health Effects of Plutonium and Radium, W.S.S. Jee, Ed. J.W. Press, Univ. of Utah, Salt Lake City, 343-362 (1976).
10. Müller, W.A., A. Luz, Influence of spatial and temporal dose distribution on bone tumour induction after incorporation of osteotropic alpha-emitting radionuclides in mice. Rep. on Third European IRPA Congress, Amsterdam 1975.
11. Rosenblatt, L.S., N.H. Hetherington, M. Goldman, L.K. Bustad, Evaluation of tumour incidence following exposure to internal emitters by application of the logistic dose-response surface. Health Phys. 21, 869-875 (1971).
12. Sacher, G.A., The Gompertz transformation in the study of the injury-mortality relationship: Application to late radiation effects and ageing. In: Radiation and Ageing, Eds. P.J. Lindop and G.J. Sacher, p. 217, Taylor and Francis, London 1966.
13. Svoboda, V., V. Kofránek, Response of femoral and vertebral colony-forming units to ^{226}Ra internal contamination in mice. Rad.Research 64, 467-474 (1975).

The dependence of late effects in mice on the temporal distribution of skeletal α-doses from ^{224}Ra and ^{227}Ra*

A. Lutz, W.A. Müller, W. Gösner, O. Hug
Institut für Biologie
Gesellschaft für Strahlen- und Umweltforschung mbH
D-8042 Neuherberg / Federal Republic of Germany

ABSTRACT

A survey is given of the long-term experiments and dosimetric studies, which have been performed during the last 10 years. All data presented refer to female NMRI mice 4 weeks old at the start of the experiment. Their mean spontaneous osteosarcoma incidence is 0.7%. Osteosarcomas of the jaws were excluded from the evaluation or considered separately. The radionuclides were injected intraperitoneally as isotonic solutions.

Dosimetric data for ^{224}Ra (half-life 3.64 days): 1 μCi/kg results in a mean skeletal dose of about 30 rad. The maximum dose rate to the skeleton is 12 rad/day. In case of repeated injections with a time interval of 3.5 days the dose rate per μCi/kg increases by a factor of 1.5.

After single injection of 1 μCi ^{224}Ra/kg up to 50 μCi/kg the osteosarcoma incidence ranges from 7 to 20% without clear mathematical function of dose dependence.

Fractionated application of ^{224}Ra was made by repeated injections every 3.5 days. The maximum osteosarcoma incidences observed in this series were 84% (total mean skeletal dose 2160 rad, maximum dose rate 24 rad/day, treatment period

* In association with EURATOM (contract No. 218-76-1 BIO D).

24 weeks) and 93% (total mean skeletal dose 1080 rad, maximum dose rate 8 rad/day, treatment period 36 weeks; i.e. about 9 months).

Dosimetric data for ^{227}Th (half-life 18.7 days): 1 μCi/kg results in a mean skeletal dose of about 200 rad. The maximum dose rate to the skeleton is 4.7 rad/day, reached about one week after injection. In case of repeated injections with a time interval of 14 days the dose rate per μCi/kg increases by a factor of about 3.0.

After single injection of ^{227}Th the maximum osteosarcoma incidence occurred at a mean skeletal dose level of about 1000-1200 rad and showed a hitherto unexplained variation between about 40 and 60%.

Comparison of the effects of ^{227}Th and its daughter product ^{223}Ra (half-life 11.4 days) at the levels of about 1200 and 2400 rad mean skeletal dose reveals a considerably lower bone tumor risk for ^{223}Ra.

Protracted application of the total dose 1000 rad over 9 months by injection of 0.28 μCi ^{227}Th/kg every two weeks resulted in an osteosarcoma incidence of about 80%.

INTRODUCTION

Late effects of ^{224}Ra - mainly the bone tumor risk - were studied in Neuherberg since 1966.

With regard to the general viewpoint of the internal irradiation risk the studies were extended to the effects of the short-lived ^{227}Th and its daughter product ^{223}Ra. Details of the experiments with ^{224}Ra and ^{227}Th have been published elsewhere (1-4).

MATERIALS AND METHODS

This report deals with the osteosarcoma induction in female NMRI mice. The animals were about four weeks old at the start of the experiments. The radionuclides were injected intraperitoneally as isotonic solutions. Each dose group and each control group included about 50 mice or more. Autopsy and X-ray examination were performed on all dead or moribund sacrified animals. Only tumors detectable on the X-ray picture were used for the statistical evaluation. Osteosarcomas of the jaws were excluded from the evaluation or considered separately. Morphological data as well as a special dose dependence of the incidence of these tumors indicate that they are not applicable to non-rodents.

For the evaluation of the tumor risk the following terms were used: 'Tumor incidence' means the total number of animals with osteosarcoma calculated as percentage of the total number of the animals at start of the experiment. The 'tumor rate' means the number of animals that died or were sacrificed with osteosarcoma during a certain time period of the experiment, calculated as percentage of the number of the surviving animals at the beginning of this time period. We calculated it for 3 months periods. The tumor rate has been calculated only, if there were at least 10 surviving animals. The term 'mortality rate' is used analogous to the tumor rate for the rate of all dead animals.

To give some rough impression of the validity of the results in groups with a different number of animals at risk, we used the 95% confidence limits, calculated for a binomial distribution.

RESULTS AND DISCUSSION

The spontaneous incidence of osteosarcomas in female NMRI mice has a mean value lower than 1%.

In mice injected activity of 1 μCi ^{224}Ra/kg results in a mean skeletal dose of about 30 rad. The maximum mean dose rate to the skeleton is 12 rad/day (5). In case of repeated injections with a time interval of 3.5 days the dose rate per μCi/kg increases by a factor 1.5.

After one single injection of ^{224}Ra (Figure 1), the osteosarcoma incidence was significantly elevated at the lowest

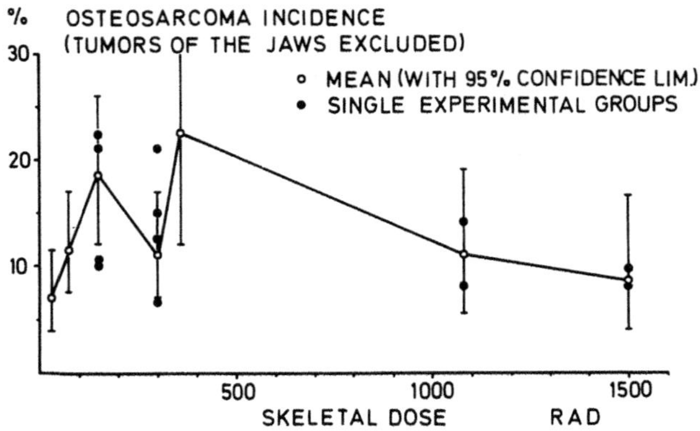

FIGURE 1

Osteosarcoma incidence (tumors of the jaws excluded) as function of mean skeletal dose after one single injection of ^{224}Ra in female NMRI mice.

dose tested, i.e. 30 rad. The incidence ranged from about 10 to 20% up to the dose group with 1500 rad. There is no clear mathematical function of the dose dependence after a single injection of ^{224}Ra.

Experiments with repeated injections of ^{224}Ra showed, that protraction of the internal irradiation period may influence considerably the efficiency of a certain internal alpha irradiation dose to the skeleton. For example this is demonstrated by experiments with a total skeletal dose of about 1100 rad (Figures 2 and 3). Single injection of the total activity was compared with fractionated application of ^{224}Ra. Repeated injections were applied every 3.5 days. The duration of treatment ranges between 4 weeks and 36 weeks. In Figure 4 is to be seen the increasing skeletal dose in the groups with a single injection, 4 weeks, 12 weeks and 36 weeks treatment. In Figure 2 the corresponding osteosarcoma incidence is shown as a function of the length of the treatment period or - in other terms - as a function of the number of injections. This corresponds to a demonstration of the increasing incidence as a function of the decreasing skeletal dose rate, since the total dose is the same for all experimental groups. The skeletal dose rates written

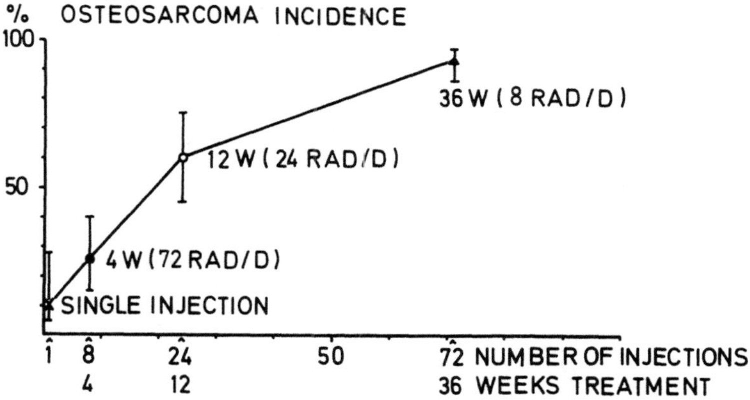

FIGURE 2

Osteosarcoma incidence (tumors of the jaws excluded) after single and fractionated (every 3.5 days) application of 36 µCi ^{224}Ra/kg (total mean skeletal dose 1080 rad) in female NMRI mice vs. number of injections or weeks treatment period.

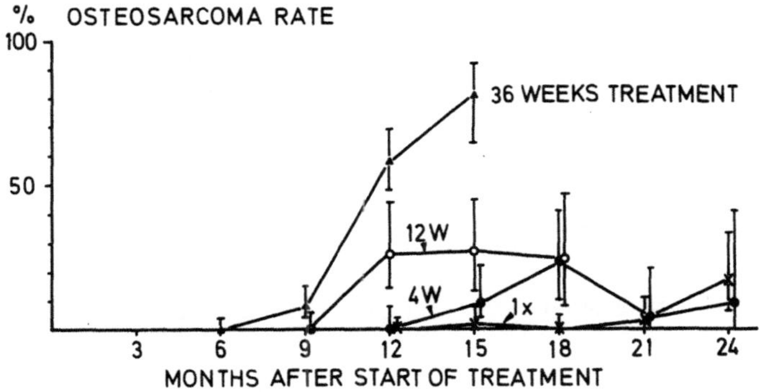

FIGURE 3

36 µCi ^{224}Ra/kg (total mean skeletal dose 1080 rad), female NMRI mice. Osteosarcoma rate vs. time after start of experiments with one single injection and fractionated (every 3.5 days) application. Treatment periods 4 weeks, 12 weeks and 36 weeks.

down by the side of the curve are maximum mean skeletal dose rates. Figure 3 shows the time function of the osteosarcoma rate for the different experimental groups. From Figure 2 it is evident that at the same dose level the highest osteosarcoma incidence, i.e. 93%, was seen in the group with the lowest maximum dose rate (8 rad/day) and the longest duration of the treatment period of about 9 months. As seen in Figure 3 in this low-dose-rate-group the osteosarcoma rate rises very steep immediately after the end of the injection period.

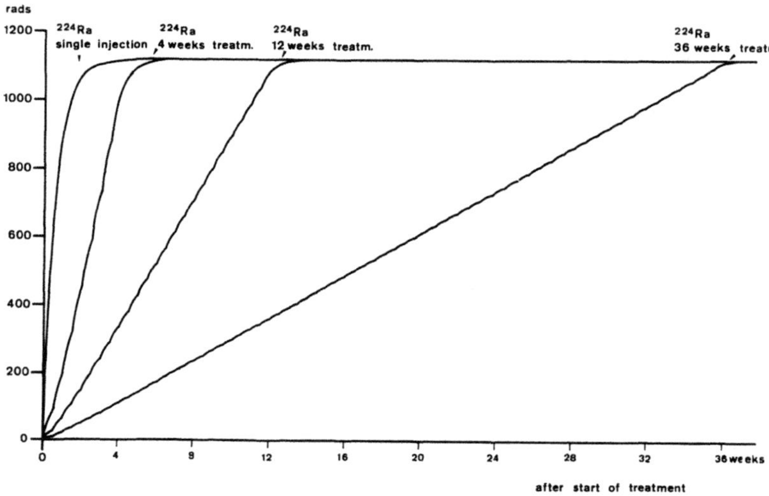

FIGURE 4

Mean skeletal dose vs. time after start of experiments with single and fractionated application of 36 µCi ^{224}Ra/kg (total mean skeletal dose 1080 rad), female NMRI mice. Treatment periods 4 weeks, 12 weeks and 36 weeks.

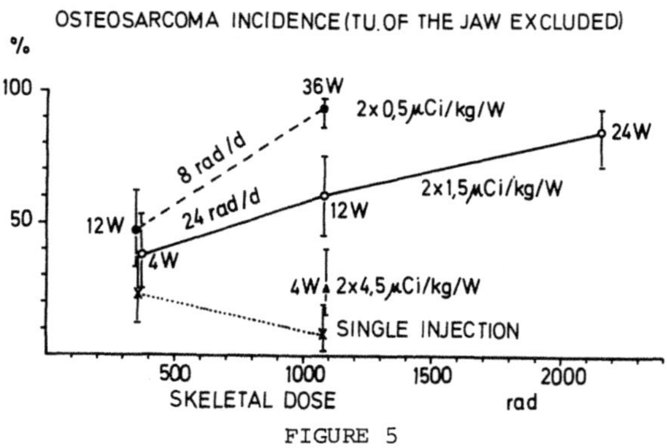

FIGURE 5

Osteosarcoma incidence (tumors of the jaws excluded) vs. total mean skeletal dose in experiments with one single injection of ^{224}Ra and fractionated application of ^{224}Ra (two injections per week) at different levels of maximum skeletal dose rate, female NMRI mice.

Figure 5 summarizes the results of all our experiments with fractionated injection of ^{224}Ra twice weekly. Here the dose dependence of the osteosarcoma incidence is clear, if we consider separately experiments with a certain level of maximum dose rate, i.e. a certain amount of activity for individual fractions of injection. For comparison the results of a single injection are drawn in the dotted curve. If one compares the points in vertical direction the increasing tumor risk can be seen again by dose protraction. But it is also obvious, that this protraction effect is in addition dose dependent. The protraction effect is much more impressive at the 1080 rad level than at the 360 rad level. At the 360 rad level the difference between the 24 rad/day group and the 8 rad/day group is not significant.

To have some more insight into the internal irradiation risk we investigated the alpha-emitting 227Th, which in contrast to ^{224}Ra belongs to the so-called bone-surface-seeking radionuclides. The half-life is 18.7 days. The half-life of its daughter product ^{223}Ra is 11.3 days. Since ^{227}Th is injected free from its daughter products the resulting time function of the dose rate in the skeleton (Figure 6) shows its maximum value about 1 week after injection. The injection of 1 µCi/kg results in a maximum skeletal dose rate of 4.7 rad/day and a total mean skeletal dose of 200 rad (6). After a single injection of ^{227}Th the osteosarcoma

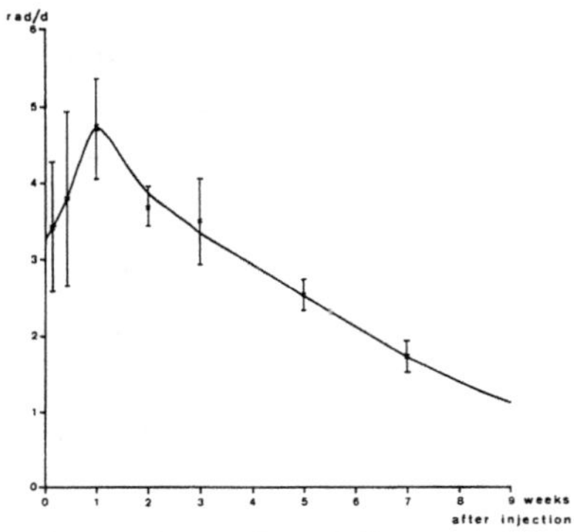

FIGURE 6

Mean skeletal dose rate (rad/day) vs. time after i.p. injection (weeks) of 1 µCi ^{227}Th/kg, female NMRI mice.

incidence is evidently dose dependent (Figure 7). We have to consider that - as compared to ^{224}Ra - the internal irradiation from ^{227}Th is more protracted, caused by the longer physical half-life. For the same total skeletal dose the maximum dose rate after a single injection of ^{227}Th is only about 5% of that in the corresponding ^{224}Ra experiment.

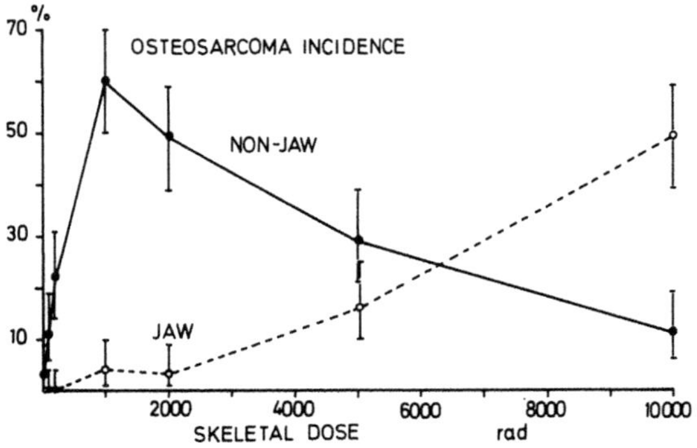

FIGURE 7

Osteosarcoma incidence in the jaws and the non-jaw skeleton vs. mean skeletal dose after one single injection of ^{227}Th, female NMRI mice.

The incidence of the non-jaw osteosarcomas had a maximum value of 60% at 1000 rad mean skeletal dose. (This maximum value of the osteosarcoma incidence after single injection of ^{227}Th showed a high range of variation in later experiments at a similar dose level. The lowest value observed was about 40%. Since we have no full explanation for this phenomenon we planned to repeat some experiments with ^{227}Th during the next year). In the higher dose groups the tumor incidence decreased. In the dose group 10 000 rad we observed mostly osteonecrosis. The lowest dose tested, i.e. 20 rad, resulted in 3% bone tumors. This value was also observed during the last ten years in a control group. For comparison the dashed curve shows the contrasting dose function of the jaw tumors.

The comparison of the effects of ^{227}Th and its volume-seeking daughter product ^{223}Ra gives some additional insight into the role of spatial and temporal distribution of dose.

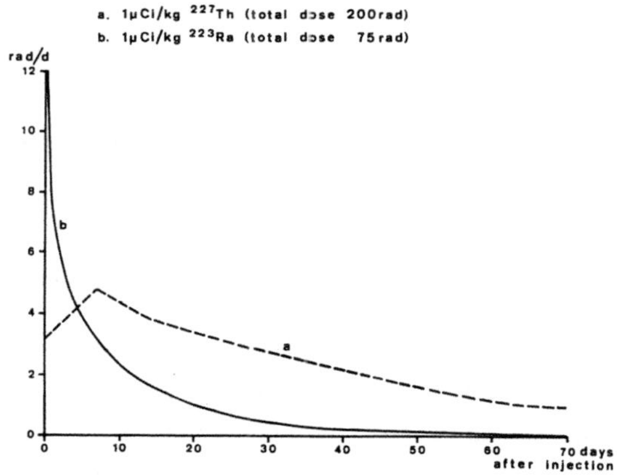

FIGURE 8

Mean skeletal dose rate (rad/day) vs. time after i.p. injection (weeks) of
a) 1 µCi ^{227}Th/kg (total mean skeletal dose 200 rad), dashed curve and
b) 1 µCi ^{223}Ra/kg (total mean skeletal dose 75 rad), female NMRI mice.

In Figure 8 one can see the very different time function of the skeletal dose rate for ^{227}Th (dashed curve) and ^{223}Ra. One has to consider that the comparison of dose rate in this diagram is done on the basis of injected µCi/kg. On the basis of the same skeletal dose, the maximum dose rate for ^{223}Ra is by a factor of more than 6 higher than after ^{227}Th incorporation. As demonstrated in Figure 9 the osteosarcoma

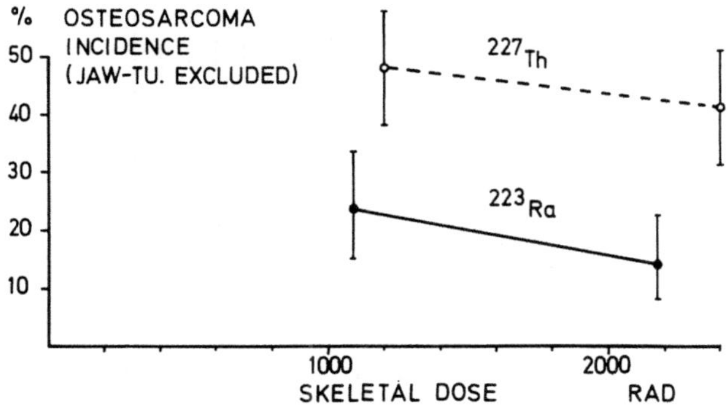

FIGURE 9

Osteosarcoma incidence (tumors of the jaws excluded) vs. skeletal dose in experiments with one single injection of ^{227}Th (dashed curve) or ^{223}Ra.

incidence per skeletal dose - tested at the level of about 1100-1200 rad and about 2300-2400 rad - is lower for ^{223}Ra. It may be not significantly different from the maximum values of 20% observed in the experiments with a single injection of ^{224}Ra. The maximum dose rate after a single injection of ^{224}Ra is about 40% of that after a ^{224}Ra injection with the corresponding total skeletal dose.

Finally it might be interesting to compare the effects of protracted internal alpha-irradiation in experiments with ^{227}Th and ^{224}Ra at a similar mean skeletal dose level of about 1000 rad and a treatment period of about 9 months. Figures 10 and 11 show the different time-function of the dose rate for both nuclides. In the ^{224}Ra experiment (dashed curve) there are the twice weekly peaks of 8 rad/day, while in the ^{227}Th experiment with injection every two weeks the dose rate increases very slowly, reaches 4 rad/day after 10 weeks and a maximum value of about 4.5 rad/day 32 weeks after the start of the treatment. The per μCi value of maximum dose rate is by a factor of more than 3 higher than after only one injection. The decrease of the dose rate after the last injection of 0.28 μCi $^{227}Th/kg$ is considerably slower than in the ^{224}Ra experiment.

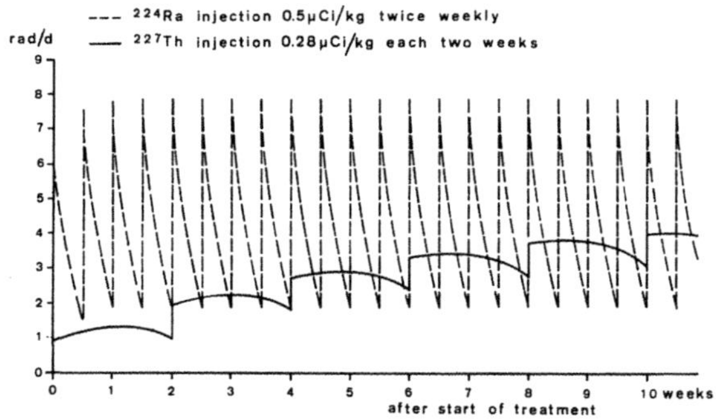

FIGURE 10

Mean skeletal dose rate (rad/day) vs. time after start of the injection period with fractionated application of ^{224}Ra and ^{227}Th in female NMRI mice.

a) 0.5 μCi $^{224}Ra/kg$ twice weekly (every 3.5 days), total amount 36 μCi/kg, total mean skeletal dose 1080 rad, dashed curve

B) 0.28 μCi $^{227}Th/kg$ every two weeks, total amount 5 μCi/kg, total mean skeletal dose 1000 rad.

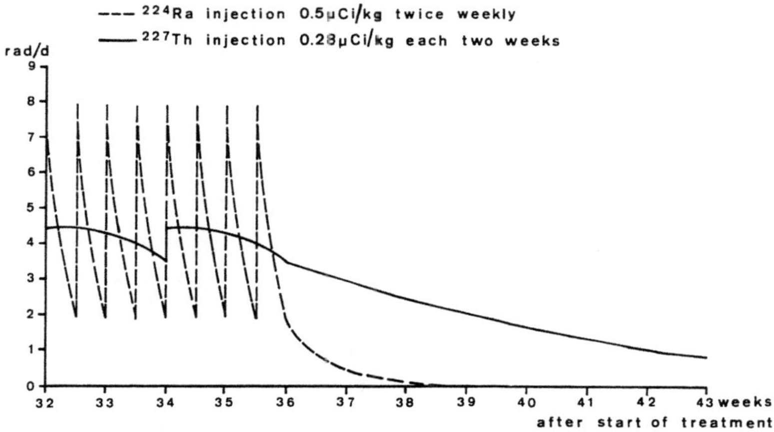

FIGURE 11

End of the curve in Figure 10.

In Figure 12 the osteosarcoma rate and the osteosarcoma incidence for both experiments is seen. There is no significant difference in the final tumor incidence for these different time schedules of internal alpha-irradiation.

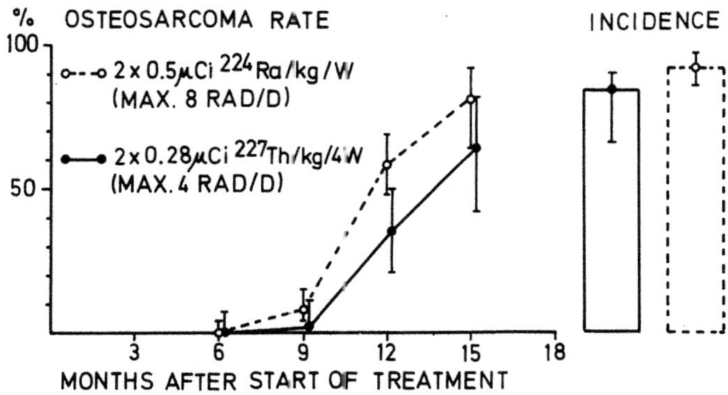

FIGURE 12

Osteosarcoma rate vs. time after start of injection period and osteosarcoma incidence (tumors of the jaws excluded) in the two experiments with fractionated application of ^{224}Ra and ^{227}Th, demonstrated in Figures 10 and 11.

The increased osteosarcoma risk by protracted internal alpha-irradiation in our experiment confirms the data from

^{224}Ra patients already published by Spiess and Mays (7).

Dvořák et al. (8) and Kofránek et al. (9) also studied the osteosarcoma induction after repeated injections of ^{224}Ra. Female ICR mice received decreasing amounts of ^{224}Ra twice weekly over 75 weeks. Comparison on the basis of total activity applied and maximum amount of single injection showed a lower osteosarcomogenic effect in ICR mice as compared to NMRI-Neuherberg mice. Spontaneous osteosarcoma incidence is not significantly different in both strains.

In connection with the proposal of Mays (10) to use data from repeated injections of ^{224}Ra as a model to predict the effects of ^{239}Pu it might be interesting to note, that the maximum incidence per dose unit in our ^{224}Ra experiment with dose rate 8 rad/day is very similar to that in Miriam Finkel's results after ^{239}Pu incorporation in CF-1 mice (11, 12). In Miriam Finkel's experiments the maximum osteosarcomogenic effectiveness was observed in the group with 77% osteosarcoma cases and 560 rad mean skeletal dose (for dose calculation see: 12) i.e. 1375 cases/10^6/rad. The maximum effectiveness per dose unit in our dose protraction experiments was achieved in the group with 47% osteosarcoma cases and mean skeletal dose 360 rad applied with maximum dose rate 8 rad/day, i.e. 1306 cases/10^6/rad.

Comparison of the results of different dose-time-schedules after fractionated application of ^{224}Ra and ^{227}Th do not indicate the need for an initial higher dose rate for bone tumor induction.

ACKNOWLEDGMENTS

We should like to thank Margit Miszkup, Kunigunde Böll, Eva de Fries, Utz Linzner, Anna Nickl, Aloisia Schneid and Joachim Wiebe for their valuable assistance in these long-term studies. We also thank Waltraud Pedit and Günter Goddeng for their assistance in preparing the manuscript.

REFERENCES

1. Hug, O., W. Gössner, W.A. Müller, A. Luz and B. Hindringer, Production of osteosarcomas in mice and rats by incorporation of Radium-224. In 'Radiation-Induced Cancer' (Proc.Symp. Athens, 1969) pp. 393-409. IAEA, Vienna 1969.
2. Müller, W.A., W. Gössner, O. Hug and A. Luz, Late effects after incorporation of the short-lived α-emitters ^{224}Ra and ^{227}Th in mice. Health Phys. - in press.
3. Gössner, W., O. Hug, A. Luz and W.A. Müller, Experimental induction of bone tumors by short-lived bone-seeking radionuclides. In 'Recent Results in Cancer Research', Vol. 54, pp. 36-49. Springer, Berlin-Heidelberg-New York, 1976.
4. Luz, A., W.A. Müller, W. Gössner and O. Hug, Estimation of tumour risk at low dose from experimental results after incorporation of short-lived bone-seeking alpha emitters ^{224}Ra and ^{227}Th in mice. In "Biological and Environmental Effects of Low-Level Radiation' (Proc. Symp. Chicago, 1975), Vol. II, pp. 171-181. IAEA, Vienna, 1976.
5. Müller, W.A., Studies on short-lived internal α-emitters in mice and rats. Part. I. ^{224}Ra. Int.J.Radiat.Biol. 20, 27-38 (1971).
6. Müller, W.A., Studies on short-lived internal α-emitters in mice and rats. Part. II. ^{227}Th. Int.J.Radiat.Biol. 20, 233-243 (1971).
7. Spiess, H. and C.W. Mays, Bone cancers induced by ^{224}Ra Th X) in children and adults. Health Phys. 19, 713-729 (1970).
8. Dvořák, V., V. Kofránek, I. Malátová, D. Bubeníková, V. Klener and V. Svoboda, Osteogenic sarcomas in mice after ^{224}Ra or ^{226}Ra administrations. Proceedings, Second International Symposium 'Biological Effects of Ra-224', München-Neuherberg, September 20-21, 1976.
9. Kofránek, V., V. Dvořák, V. Klener, A. Sedlák, V. Svoboda, D. Bubeníková, Z. Onyskowová, J. Thomas, V. Lenger and J. Salava, Biological effects of ^{224}Ra and ^{226}Ra and

their relative radiotoxicity in mice. Proceedings Second International Symposium 'Biological Effects of Ra-224', München-Neuherberg, September 20-21, 1976.

10. Mays, C.W., Estimated risk from ^{239}Pu to human bone, liver and lung. Health Phys. 19, 373-380 (1970).

11. Finkel, M.P. and B.O. Biskis, Toxicity of Plutonium in mice. Health Phys. 8, 565-579 (1962).

12. Mays, C.W. and R.D. Lloyd, Bone sarcoma incidence vs. alpha particle dose. In 'Radiobiology of Plutonium' (Stover, B.J. and W.S.S. Jee, Eds.), pp. 409-430. The J.W. Press, Dept. Anatomy, Univ. Utah, Salt Lake City, 1972.

Histopathology of early effects of ^{224}Ra on bone tissue*

K.-H. Marquart and W. Bössner

Department of General and Experimental Pathology,
Institute of Biology,
Gesellschaft für Strahlen- und Umweltforschung mbH München,
D-8042 Neuherberg, Federal Republic of Germany

ABSTRACT

Early morphologic changes in the proximal tibial metaphysis of ^{224}Ra-treated rats and mice are presented. The methods for the investigations performed include autoradiography, histology, enzyme histochemistry, and electron microscopy.

Autoradiographs showed high concentration of ^{224}Ra in the active ossification zone beneath the epiphyseal cartilage. During 90 days following ^{224}Ra administration (between 10 and 300 μCi/kg), radiation-induced lesions occurred in epiphyseal cartilage and primary spongiosa of rates resulting in severe disturbance of endochondral ossification. Depending on the amounts of ^{224}Ra injected, a more or less complete loss of alkaline phosphatase in cartilage cells and osteoblasts was found. The acid phosphatase content was not markedly affected. Studies on the cell population in osteogenic tissue of mice showed a marked reduction of osteoblasts and mesenchymal cells in the first 2 weeks after the incorporation of 25 or 75 μCi/kg of ^{224}Ra.

Electron microscopic examinations revealed alterations in all cell types of the trabecular bone tissue of mice

* In association with EURATOM (Contract No. 218-76-1 BIO D).

already 2 hours after the incorporation of 1.5 μCi/kg of ^{224}Ra. The ultrastructural changes consisted of chromatin condensations in the nuclei, various damages in the mitochondria, dilatation of the endoplasmic reticulum, and vacuolation of the Golgi complex. The mitochondria appeared to be the cellular organelles most sensitive to the effects of ^{224}Ra administration. The early ultrastructural changes in bone cells of the proximal tibial metaphysis are regarded as the result of direct alpha-radiation upon the cells.

In order to obtain information about the morphology of early effects of ^{224}Ra on bone tissue, autoradiographic, histologic, histochemical, and electron microscopic investigations were performed. We studied the trabecular bone tissue of the proximal tibial metaphysis of ^{224}Ra-treated Wistar rats and NMRI mice. It was of interest to learn the sequence of histopathologic bone changes following the incorporation of ^{224}Ra. Further, we wanted to know which of the bone cells and which of the cellular organelles were most sensitive to the alpha-emitting radionuclide.

More data than in the present report as well as details of the materials and methods used for the experiments have been published in earlier papers (1-5).

Few hours after the incorporation of ^{224}Ra, autoradiographs showed a high concentration of alpha-tracks in the active ossification zone beneath the epiphyseal cartilage of the tibia of rats and mice. A concentration of alpha-tracks was also seen in the epiphysis, whereas only few tracks were found in the epiphyseal cartilage.

From 1 to 90 days following a single intraperitoneal injection of ^{224}Ra amounts between 10 and 300 μCi/kg, radiation-induced lesions occurred in epiphyseal cartilage and primary spongiosa of rats resulting in severe disturbance of endochondral ossification. After administration of ^{224}Ra, the epiphyseal cartilage plate was enlarged and showed an irregularly formed metaphyseal border. The length of columns of proliferating flattened cartilage cells diminished markedly, whereas hypertrophic cartilage cells near the zone of ossification increased and were enlarged. These cells frequently showed regressive alterations, and spots of asbestos-like degeneration developed in the cartilage matrix. After about 1 week, irregularly shaped portions of the hypertrophic cartilage began to be penetrated and substituted by proliferating connective tissue which accompanied invading blood vessels. Later, this tissue differentiated into or was substituted by osteogenic tissue. Osteoblasts in the primary spongiosa began to decrease after the first few days, while osteoclasts seemed to diminish only in the higher dose levels. The intertrabecular haematopoietic tissue within the metaphysis was completely destroyed, and within 8 days, peritrabecular fibrosis developed.

The described histologic changes appeared in the tissue parallel to characteristic alterations of the enzyme content. Depending on the amounts of ^{224}Ra injected, a more or less complete loss of alkaline phosphatase in cartilage cells and osteoblasts was found. The acid phosphatase content was not so markedly affected. Chondroclasts, osteoclasts and reticular cells still retained their enzyme content also in the higher dose levels.

Additionally to the described findings in the rat tibia, quantitative studies on the cell population in the proximal tibial metaphysis of mice were performed. These studies showed a marked reduction of osteoblasts and mesenchymal cells in the first 2 weeks following administration of 25 or 75 μCi/kg of ^{224}Ra. In the third week after 25 μCi/kg, the numbers of cells reached nearly the control values, while the repopulation of the metaphysis by bone cells was not yet finished at that time after 75 μCi/kg. The numbers of osteoclasts and osteocytes did not differ significantly after ^{224}Ra administration from the control values.

Electron microscopic investigations revealed alterations in all types of bone cells of the proximal tibial metaphysis of mice already 2 hours after the incorporation of 1.5 μCi/kg of ^{224}Ra. Table I shows the various experimental groups of mice used for electron microscopic study of tibial trabecular bone tissue. The ultrastructural cellular changes consisted mainly of chromatin condensations in the nuclei, various

TABLE I

GROUPS OF MICE SACRIFICED AT SHORT TIME INTERVALS AFTER THE INCORPORATION OF SMALL AMOUNTS OF ^{224}RA

Group of mice	Incorporated amount of ^{224}Ra (μCi/kg of body weight)	Time interval between the injection of ^{224}Ra and sacrifice of the mice
I	1	24 hours
II	1	5 days
III	1.5	2 hours
IV	5	24 hours
V	5	5 days

damages in the mitochondria, dilatation of the rough endoplasmic reticulum, and vacuolation of the Golgi complex.

Two hours, 24 hours and 5 days after incorporation of the small amounts of ^{224}Ra, the chromatin in the nuclei of many bone cells was partially condensed, mainly in the marginal zone. Additionally, the perinuclear space was enlarged (Figure 1).

Completely pyknotic or karyolytic nuclei of bone cells appeared at a period later than 2 hours following ^{224}Ra administration. Such nuclei were found both 24 hours and 5 days after either 1 or 5 μCi/kg of ^{224}Ra.

Nuclear damage was found in all bone cell types of the metaphysis, also in osteoclasts which, on the light microscopic level, seemed to be more radioresistant than osteoblasts.

Cells showing damages in their nuclei always showed alterations in other cellular organelles. The most frequently observed changes following ^{224}Ra incorporation occurred in the mitochondria. These were often the only cellular changes which were to be seen. Alterations in mitochondria consisted of partial to nearly complete loss of mitochondrial cristae, swelling, and dissociation or disruption of both limiting mitochondrial membranes (Figure 2).

Additonally, elongated giant mitochondria, up to 3-4 times the size of normal oval-formed ones, were sometimes found in bone cells after ^{224}Ra administration.

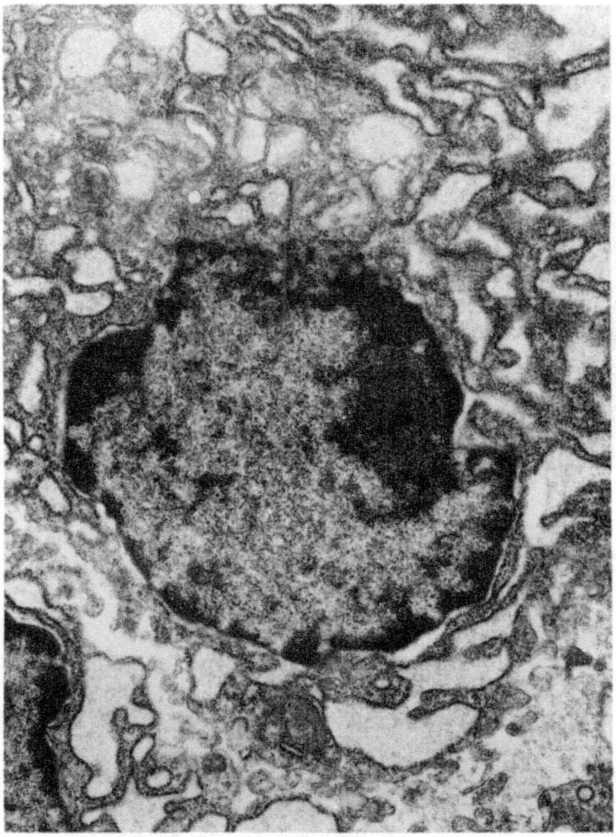

FIGURE 1

Electron micrograph of a portion of an osteoblast from the proximal tibial metaphysis of a mouse. The animal was sacrificed 24 hr after the incorporation of 5 μCi/kg of ^{224}Ra. The nucleus of the bone cell shows a marginal zone of condensed chromatin. The perinuclear space is partially enlarged. The rough endoplasmic reticulum and the Golgi complex (in the upper part of the picture) are dilated and form large cisternae. X 20,000.

Normally, the membranes of the rough endoplasmic reticulum in osteoblasts and osteocytes were arranged in almost parallel rows. After incorporation of ^{224}Ra, the tubular elements of the endoplasmic reticulum in many osteoblasts and osteocytes were dilated and formed cisternae of various sizes (Figures 1 and 3).

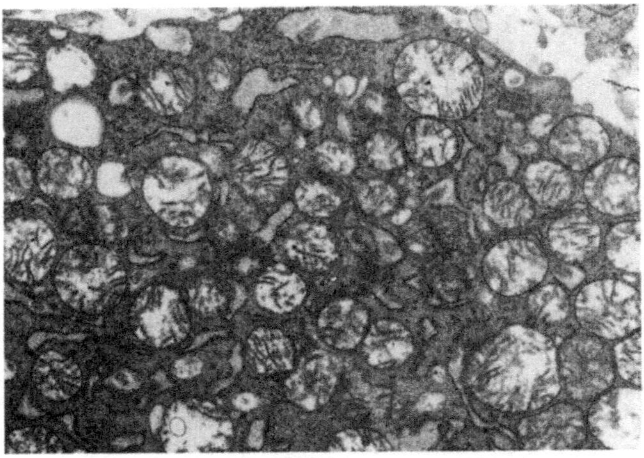

FIGURE 2

Swollen mitochondria with partial cristolysis in an osteoclast 24 hrs following the administration of 5 µCi/kg of ^{224}Ra. X 15,000.

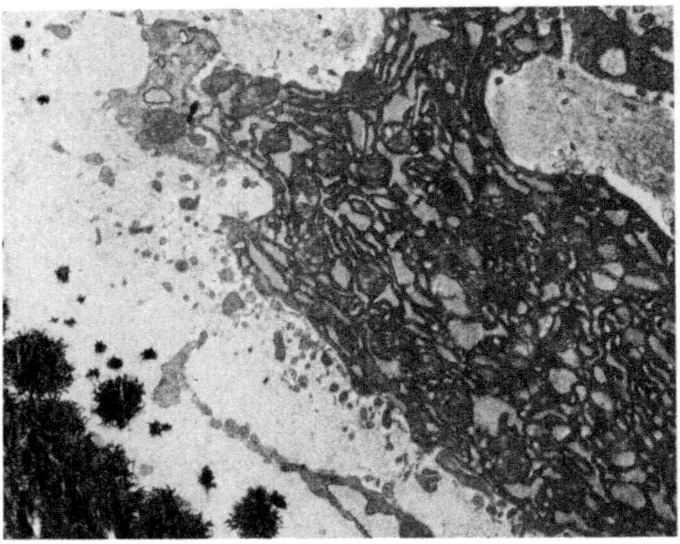

FIGURE 3

Osteoblast, 24 hrs after 5 µCi/kg of ^{224}Ra, showing dilated rough endoplasmic reticulum. The bone cell is surrounded by collagen fibrils and mineralized bone matrix (in the lower part of the picture). X 10,000.

These alterations were found only in cells showing changes in mitochondrial and nuclear structure. Occasionally, the tubular and vesicular elements of the Golgi complex in bone cells were dilated after administration of ^{224}Ra (Figures 1 and 4).

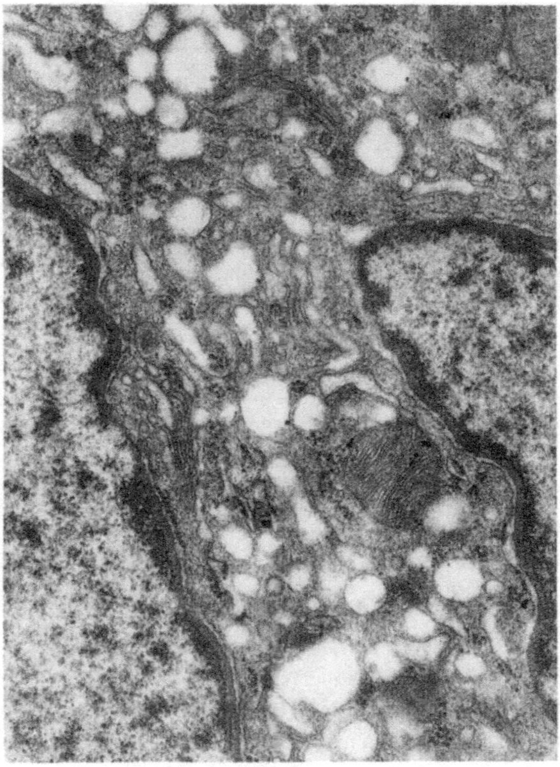

FIGURE 4

Vacuolated Golgi complex in an osteoclast 24 hrs after 1 μCi/kg of ^{224}Ra. Portions of two nuclear profiles are visible. X 30,000.

Endothelial cells of some capillaries within the tibial metaphysis of ^{224}Ra-treated mice contained an osmiophilic cytoplasm and damaged mitochondria (Figure 5). The endothelial wall of sinusoids was often ruptured and red blood cells could be seen in the extravasal space.

Our studies showed that early ultrastructural changes were present in all bone cell types of the proximal tibial

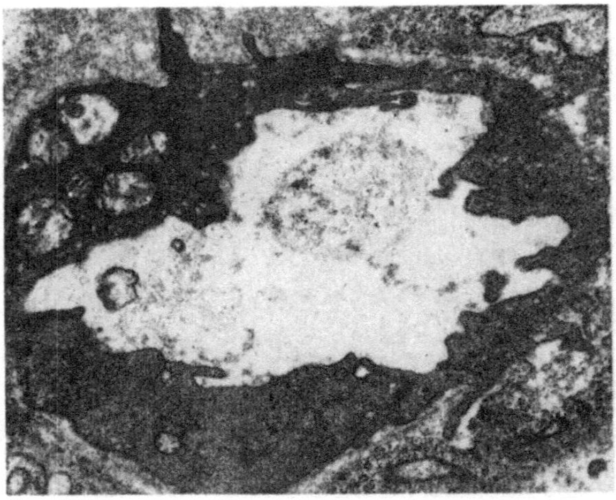

FIGURE 5

Cross-sectioned capillary from the tibial metaphysis 24 hrs after the incorporation of 5 μCi/kg ^{224}Ra. The endothelium displays electron-dense cytoplasm and damaged mitochondria. X 15,000.

metaphysis of mice after incorporation of ^{224}Ra. The mitochondria appeared to be the cellular organelles most sensitive to the effects of ^{224}Ra administration. The observed giant mitochondria were presumably the morphological expression of a cellular process trying to compensate for damaged mitochondria by the hypertrophy of others.

It is thought that all cellular changes resulted from the effects of direct alpha-radiation emitted from the incorporated ^{224}Ra which was diffusely deposited in the trabecular mineralized bone matrix surrounding the cells. The alterations are similar to those reported in cells from various tissues of different species after local or total-body X-irradiation (6-8).

The significance of ^{224}Ra-induced early ultrastructural changes in trabecular bone tissue of mice remains to be clarified, especially in relation to late effects of ^{224}Ra. At present, only few information is available about the initial events preceding the development of radionuclide-induced osteosarcomas. We have started electron microscopic studies in the latency period of ^{224}Ra bone tumors which perhaps will provide further information.

REFERENCES

1. Gössner, W. and M. Schwabe, Histochemische Untersuchungen am Knochen nach Inkorporation von Ra-224 (Thorium-X). Verh.Dtsch.Ges.Path. 52, 334-338 (1968).
2. Gössner, W., Grundlagen und allgemeine pathologische Anatomie der Strahlenschäden. Verh.Dtsch.Ges.Path. 56, 168-187 (1972).
3. Becker, G., C. Lepp, H. Pömsl and A. Luz, Störung des Knochenwachstums nach Incorporation von Ra-224 (Thorium-X) bei der Maus. Verh.Dtsch.Ges.Path. 56, 448-452 (1972).
4. Marquart, K.-H., Frühe Ultrastrukturveränderungen in der Tibiametaphyse der Maus nach Inkorporation von Ra-224. Verh.Dtsch.Ges.Path. 57, 466 (1973).
5. Marquart, K.-H., Early ultrastructural changes in osteocytes from the proximal tibial metaphysis of mice after the incorporation of ^{224}Ra. Radiat.Res. 69, 40-53 (1977).
6. Cottier, H., Histopathologie der Wirkung ionisierender Strahlen auf höhere Organismen (Tier und Mensch). In 'Encyclopedia of Medical Radiology' (L. Diethelm, O Olsson, F. Strnad, H. Vieten and A. Zuppinger, Eds.), Vol. II, Radiation Biology, Part 2, pp. 35-272. Springer, Berlin-Heidelberg-New York, 1966.
7. Berdjis, C.C., Cell. In 'Pathology of Irradiation' (C.C. Berdjis, Ed.), pp. 10-31. Williams & Wilkins, Baltimore, 1971.
8. Betz, E.H., Morphologische Veränderungen des lymphatischen Systems nach Bestrahlung. In 'Die Strahlenwirkung auf das Lymphsystem unter besonderer Berücksichtigung der kleinen Dosen' (K.H. Kärcher and C. Streffer, Eds.), pp. 29-36. Springer, Berlin-Heidelberg-New York, 1974.

Expression of type C RNA virus particles in ^{224}Ra-induced osteosarcomas*

V. Erfle and K.-H. Marquart

Institut für Biologie
Gesellschaft für Strahlen- und Umweltforschung mbH
D-8042 Neuherberg / Federal Republic of Germany

ABSTRACT

The experiments reported are part of a program to evaluate the role of RNA tumor viruses in radionuclide-induced osteosarcomas of mice. The expression of type C RNA virus particles was investigated in ^{224}Ra-induced primary osteosarcomas as well as in transplanted tumors and cell cultures derived from the primary osteosarcomas. Virus particle expression could be detected in primary osteosarcomas by electron microscopy as intracisternal type A and type C particles and by the simultaneous detection test as a particulate structure containing a high molecular weight RNA associated with a reverse transcriptase. The same viral markers were also detected in transplanted osteosarcomas. In contrast to tumors of inbred C3H x $101/F_1$ mice, primary and transplanted osteosarcomas in random-bred NMRI mice did not show type C virus particles by electron microscopy nor viral parameters in the simultaneous detection test. In vitro cultivated osteosarcomas from NMRI mice also produced virus particles. The virus particles possessed the typical properties of RNA tumor viruses like type C morphology, a density in sucrose of

* In association with EURATOM (Contract No. 218-76-1 BIO D).

$1,16-1,18\ g/cm^3$ and a reverse transcriptase associated with a high molecular weight RNA of 60-70 S. Thus far, no oncogenic activity of the virus particles associated with the tumors or cell cultures could be detected.

INTRODUCTION

The detection that murine leukemias are caused by a virus led to the assumption that radiation-induced leukemias in mice could be induced by radiation activation of a latent oncogenic virus. This was partially confirmed by the isolation of leukemogenic viruses from S-ray-induced leukemias in mice by Gross (1), Liebermann and Kaplan (2) and by others. Other well-known radiation-induced tumors are the radionuclide-induced osteosarcomas in man and animals (for literature see 3). In mice, osteosarcomas can also be induced by a virus, the so-called FBJ virus which was isolated by Finkel, Biskis and Jinkins (4) in 1966. The aim of our present investigations is to test whether there is a relation between viral and radiation sarcomagenesis.

The above mentioned tumor viruses belong to the type C virus group of the RNA tumor viruses. These viruses have unique properties. In the electron microscope, they have a spherical structure with a diameter of about 90-100 nm. These virus particles possess an outer shell and a concentric inner electron-dense core. The type C particles are released from the cells by a characteristic budding process. The density of the particles in sucrose is $1,16-1,18\ g/cm^3$. They exhibit two biochemical properties unique to them as a group: they possess a large single-stranded RNA molecule with a sedimentation coefficient of 60-70 S, which can be easily denatured into two 35 S subunits and several small pieces. They also contain a reverse transcriptase, an enzyme capable of using the viral RNA as a template to generate a complementary DNA copy.

In the literature there are only few reports concerning the association of radiation-induced osteosarcomas with

RNA tumor viruses. Especially, Finkel and her colleagues have presented some evidence for the association of RNA-tumor viruses with ^{90}Sr-induced bone sarcoma in mice. They were able to show type C particles in these tumors (5) as well as antibodies in ^{90}Sr bone sarcoma-bearing mice neutralising FBJ osteosarcoma virus (6). Frazier et al. (7) described the detection of a reverse transcriptase complexed to a high molecular weight RNA in Plutionium-induced osteosarcomas of dogs. Extensive studies to transmit the tumors in neonatal mice by cell-free extracts resulted in the growth of very few osteosarcomas (5).

MATERIALS AND METHODS

We have used two methods to detect expression of type C RNA virus information in primary and transplanted osteosarcomas: electron microscopy and the simultaneous detection test (8). The method of the simultaneous detection of a 70 S RNA and of a reverse transcriptase makes use of the observation that after a reverse transcriptase reaction the initial DNA product is complexed to the 70 S RNA template by hydrogen bonds. In sedimentation analysis the DNA product will be found cosedimenting with the 70 S RNA template. Therefore the detection of a DNA product complexed to a RNA with the sedimentation behaviour of the RNA of RNA tumor viruses provides evidence for the presence of a reverse transcriptase using a 70 S RNA template, and hence, for the presence of a RNA tumor virus.

The simultaneous detection method is shown in Figure 1 (9). The osteosarcoma cells were homogenised and the nuclei were removed by low-speed centrifugation. The cytoplasmic supernatant was fractioned by density centrifugation and concentrated to yield a cytoplasmic pellet containing membranes and, if present, viral particles. The pellet was treated with 0,1% Triton X-100 to disrupt possible viral particles and used in an endogenous reverse transcriptase reaction in the presence of Actinomycin D and Distamycin A

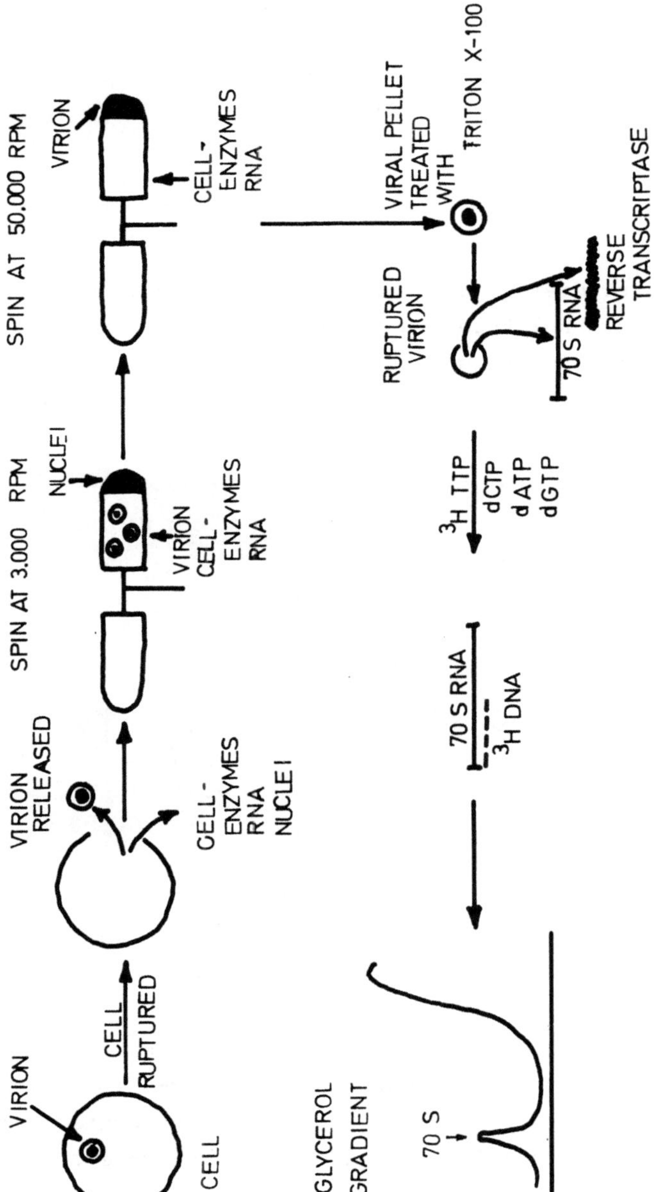

FIGURE 1

Simultaneous detection of 70 S RNA and reverse transcriptase in cells (9).

to inhibit DNA-instructed DNA synthesis. The reaction was freed from protein by phenol treatment and analyzed in a glycerol sedimentation velocity gradient. For density determination, viral particles were centrifuged overnight in a 20-60% sucrose gradient.

RESULTS

In our studies we were able to detect by electron microscopy intracisternal type A and type C particles in ^{224}Ra-induced osteosarcomas. Figure 2 shows intracisternal type A particles found in an osteoblast from an osteosarcoma of a NMRI mouse.

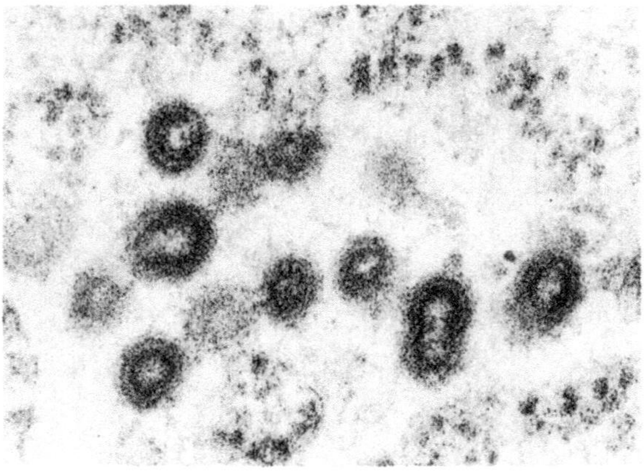

FIGURE 2

Intracisternal type A particles in an osteoblast from an osteosarcoma of a NMRI mouse. X 160,000.

The particles are spherical, have a diameter of about 80 nm, and consist of two electron-dense, ring-shaped, membraneous shells which surround an electron-lucent center. The particles occur nearly exclusively in cisternae of the rough endoplasmic reticulum.

Figure 3 shows mature type C particles in the extracellular space of an osteosarcoma of a C3H x $101/F_1$ mouse. These particles possess the typical type C morphology of

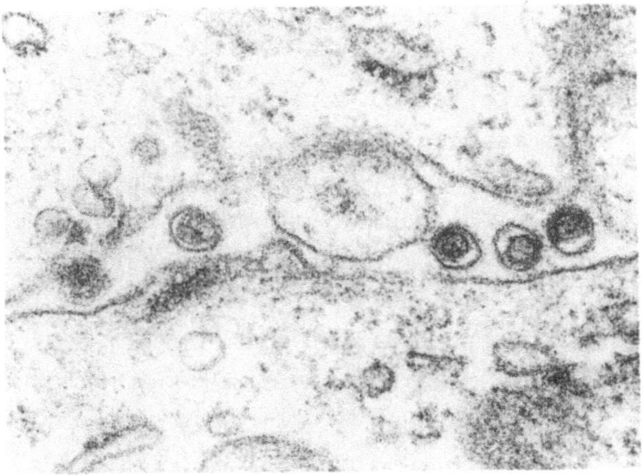

FIGURE 3

Mature type C particles in the extracellular space of an osteosarcoma of a C3H x $101/F_1$ mouse. X 80,000.

RNA tumor viruses.

These results were confirmed for C3H x $101/F_1$ osteosarcomas by simultaneous detection tests. After a reverse transcriptase reaction with cytoplasmic material of a ^{224}Ra-induced tumor, sedimentation analysis showed a ^3H-DNA radioactivity peak in the 60-70 S position of the gradient. This peak is sensitive to RNAse digestion prior to velocity sedimentation. This indicates that RNA-directed DNA synthesis has taken place on a high molecular weight RNA template of 60-70 S. It therefore can be concluded that particles are present in the osteosarcomas of C3H x $101/F_1$ mice which are similar to the RNA tumor viruses.

We have established two transplantable osteosarcoma lines, one originating from a ^{224}Ra tumor of a random-bred NMRI mouse, the other from a ^{224}Ra tumor of a F_1 hybrid mouse of the two inbred mouse strains C3H and 101. In both tumor lines, intracisternal type A particles could be detected by electron microscopy. These particles had the same appearance and morphology as those in the primary osteosarcomas. Additionally, immature and mature type C particles were found in the transplant osteosarcomas from C3H x $101/f_1$ mice.

The immature particles consisted of three electron-dense, ring-shaped shells which surrounded an electron-lucent center and had a diameter of about 100 nm.

Figure 4 shows the glycerol sedimentation of ^{3}H-DNA product and high molecular weight RNA template after a simultaneous detection test with a transplantable osteosarcoma of C3H x $101/F_1$ mice. The second peak seen here in the 35 S position of the gradient is occasionally observed and may be due to conformational changes in the 70 S RNA template. With a transplantable osteosarcoma from NMRI mice, no positive reaction could be obtained in simultaneous detection tests.

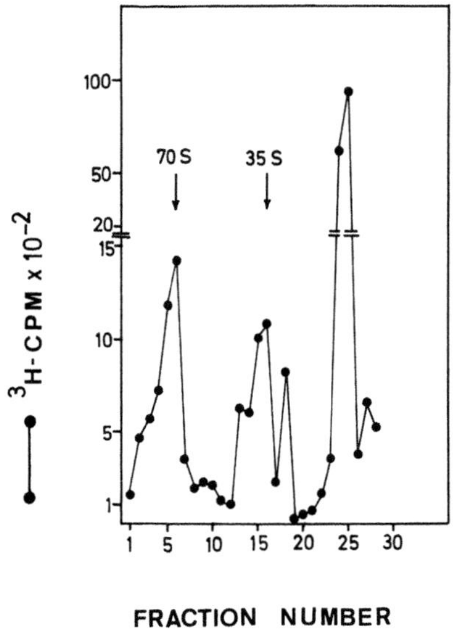

FIGURE 4

Glycerol gradient sedimentation profile of a high molecular weight RNA and tritium labelled DNA complex after simultaneous detection test with a transplanted osteosarcoma of a C3H x $101/F_1$ mouse.

To further study the expression of RNA tumor viruses in ^{224}Ra-induced osteosarcomas another series of experiments was done with in vitro cultured osteosarcomas. The tumors stemmed from NMRI as well as from C3H x $101/F_1$ mice. All established cell cultures released virus particles into the cell culture medium. The virus particles had the following properties: they were extracellular, had typical type C morphology and were released from the cell surface by budding. In addition, they possessed a density of about 1,16-1,18 g/cm^3 in sucrose gradients (Figure 5). The particles encapsulated a high molecular weight RNA with a sedimentation coefficient of about 60-70 S. Associated with the RNA was a reverse transcriptase which used the viral RNA as template for synthesis of a DNA product. The newly synthesized DNA product is complexed to a high molecular weight template RNA as shown with glycerol gradient sedimentation analysis.

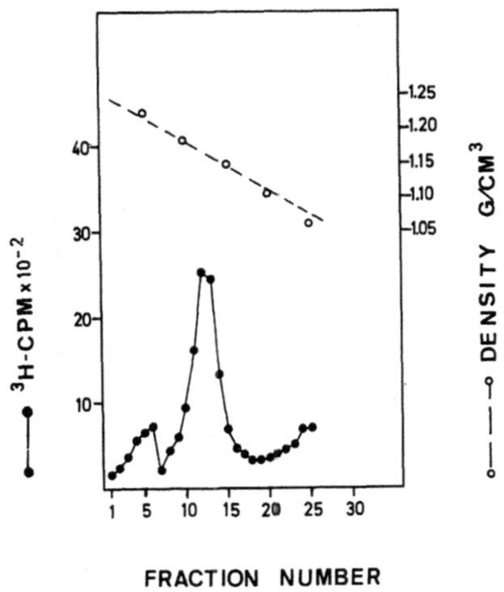

FIGURE 5

Sucrose density profile of tritium labelled virus particles from a cell culture of an osteosarcoma of a NMRI mouse.

DISCUSSION

The results presented here show that type C RNA virus particle information is expressed in primary and transplanted ^{224}Ra-induced osteosarcomas of C3H x 101/F$_1$ mice. Only after cultivation in vitro, osteosarcomas of random-bred NMRI mice as well produce type C RNA virus particles. This difference between the outbred NMRI mice and the F$_1$ hybrids of inbred

C3H and 101 mice may be due to a higher immunocompetence of the NMRI mice which may result in the suppression of virus particle-producing osteosarcoma cells.

The morphological and biochemical properties of the viral particles in osteosarcomas and their cell cultures are typical for oncogenic RNA tumor viruses. The possible oncogenicity of the expressed type C RNA virus particles was tested in newborn and adult mice with cell free extracts from induced osteosarcomas and with virus derived from osteosarcoma cell cultures. No oncogenic potential could be detected thus far with these virus particles. The virus particle expression may be the translation of endogenous type C virus information which may have no relation to the process of osteosarcomagenesis. This information may be a marker for the transformed state of the osteosarcoma cells.

But a few successful cell-free transmissions of ^{90}Sr-induced osteosarcomas in mice by Finkel et al. (5) indicate that at least in some radiation-induced osteosarcomas oncogenic type C RNA viruses are present. Whether the virus-particles expressed in ^{224}Ra osteosarcomas have no oncogenic potential or lack only a helper virus not expressed in the tumors has to be clarified by further experiments.

REFERENCES

1. Gross, L., Serial cell-free passage of a radiation-activated mouse leukemia agent. Proc.Soc.Exp.Biol.Med. 100, 102-105 (1959).
2. Lieberman, M. and H.S. Kaplan, Leukemogenic activity of filtrates from radiation-induced lymphoid tumors of mice. Science 130, 387-388 (1959).
3. Vaughan, J.J., The effects of irradiation on the skeleton. Oxford, Clarendon Press, 1973.
4. Finkel, M.P., B.O. Biskis and P.B. Jinkins, Virus induction of osteosarcomas in mice. Science 151, 698-700 (1966).
5. Finkel, M.P., C.A. Reilly Jr., B.O. Biskis and I.L. Greco,

Bone tumor viruses. In 'Bone - Certain Aspects of Neoplasia' (Price, C.H.G. and F.G.M. Ross, Eds.), pp. 353-364. Butterworths, London, 1973.

6. Reilly, C.A. Jr. and M.P. Finkel, Evidence of FBJ virus antigen in ^{90}Sr-induced osteosarcomas. Radiat.Res. 47, 252-253 (1971).

7. Frazier, M.E., J.F. Park, W.S.S. Jee and G. Taylor, RNA-instructed DNA polymerase activity in radiation-induced osteosarcomas. In 'The Health Effects of Plutonium and Radium' (Jee, W.S.S., Ed.), pp. 707-716. J.W. Press, Salt Lake City, 1976.

8. Schlom, J. and S. Spiegelman, Simultaneous detection of the reverse transcriptase and high molecular weight RNA unique to oncogenic RNA viruses. Science 174, 840-843 (1971).

9. Hehlmann, R, W. Baxt, D. Kufe and S. Spiegelman, Molecular evidence for a viral etiology of human leukemias, lymphomas, and sarcomas. Am.J.Clin.Pathol. 60, 65-79 (1973).

Bone sarcoma to man from ^{224}Ra, ^{226}Ra, and ^{239}Pu*

C.W. Mays and H. Spiess

Radiobiology Laboratory, University of Utah Medical Center
Salt Lake City, Utah, USA 84132
and
Kinderpoliklinik Universität München
München / Federal Republic of Germany

ABSTRACT

The induction of bone sarcomas increases with both dose and protraction of ^{224}Ra irradiation. From ^{224}Ra data in man, we estimate that the risk coefficient ranges from about 40 up to 200 bone sarcomas/10^6 person·rad of average skeletal dose, depending on whether the ^{224}Ra is given in a single injection or given weekly for several years. Limited experimental results in beagles and mice suggest that the risk per rad should be roughly similar for protracted skeletal irradiation from ^{239}Pu and ^{224}Ra, both of which decay to a large extent on bone surfaces. The risk coefficient for long-lived ^{226}Ra and ^{228}Ra, which decay mostly within bone volume, is much smaller, and is estimated by us to lie between 6 and 53 bone sarcomas/10^6 person·rad.

Of special interest is the risk from the ^{224}Ra therapy currently being used in Germany, of 10 weekly injections, each of 28 μCi ^{224}Ra, which gives a cumulative average skeletal dose of 56 rad to a 70 kg adult. Present data from the ^{224}Ra patients indicate that the resulting risk from induced bone sarcoma is between 0 and 0.5%.

* Supported by USERDA Contract EY-76-C-02-0119, and by EURATOM Contract 218-76-1-BIO D.

INTRODUCTION

^{224}Ra is a radium isotope whose short 3.62-day half-life (1) causes much of its α-particle decay within the skeleton to occur on bone surfaces (2-5). Following the Second World War, about 2000 German patients received repeated injections of ^{224}Ra, mainly for the treatment of tuberculosis and ankylosing spondylitis (6-11). Among the 900 traced patients in the Spiess series, 54 have developed bone sarcomas (48 with known dose and 6 with unknown dose) (11).

^{226}Ra is a radium isotope whose long half-life of 1600 years permits diffusion into the interior of the calcified bone where its α-particles are much less likely to damage cells than if emitted from bone surfaces. In several thousand American subjects, mostly radium dial painters, bone sarcomas have occurred in 82 persons (54 cases with known dose plus 28 cases with unknown dose) (12).

^{239}Pu is an α-emitter that initially deposits on bone surfaces (13, 14). At later times some of the ^{239}Pu becomes buried under layers of new bone, while some of the released ^{239}Pu redeposits back onto bone surfaces. Thus, both ^{239}Pu and ^{224}Ra decay partly on bone surfaces and partly within bone volume. This fact has led us to assume that the effects from protracted irradiation from repeated injections of ^{224}Ra in man could be used to approximate the risk from ^{239}Pu-induced bone sarcomas (15, 16). Today, in the mind of the general public, as well as the scientific community, there is more concern about the toxicity of plutonium than of any other element in the Periodic Table.

A large number of persons have been exposed occupationally to small amounts of ^{239}Pu: 'Among an estimated 16,000 people in the United States who have been employed in operations that could involve exposure to plutonium, about 5,000 have some measurable evidence of internal plutonium deposition.' (17). So far, none have developed bone sarcomas, primarily because of protective measures to minimize exposure to plutonium. But as the number of exposed persons increases and their years at risk build up, it is possible that some of these persons may develop plutonium-induced cancers of lung, liver or bone. The physical half-life of 24,000 years for ^{239}Pu and its long biological retention insures that irradiation from its internal deposition will continue throughout life.

The topics in this paper are: Skeletal dosimetry, latent periods in man, protraction effect, and bone sarcoma risk to man. In keeping with the theme of this symposium, the main emphasis will be on ^{224}Ra.

SKELETAL DOSIMETRY

For details on our calculations of dose, see Ref. (8). Based on the literature survey of Maletskos et al. (18), we assumed that the typical fraction of intravenously injected ^{224}Ra atoms decaying within the human skeleton was 60% for children 1-15 years old, 40% for adolescents 16-20 years old, and 20% for adults. We further assumed that the skeletal ^{224}Ra decayed half on bone surfaces and half within bone volume, and that the daughter products produced in the skeleton remained there. Actually, a small fraction of these daughter atoms will escape from the skeleton, but this will be opposed by skeletal deposition of some of the injected daughter atoms.

Marshall et al. (3, 4) later developed a theoretical model which predicts *for adults* that 10% of the injected ^{224}Ra decays on bone surfaces (in exact agreement with the 10% assumed by us), but that only 1.5% decays within bone volume (considerably lower than our assumed 10%). At this time, it is uncertain whether the Marshall values or ours are the most reliable, since neither was based on direct experimental data on the retention and distribution of radium in bone at short times after injection. If and when these data become available, it seems likely that both the Marshall model and our assumptions may need some revision. However, both models yield similar endosteal doses for adults injected with 1 μCi ^{224}Ra/kg (105 rad, according to Marshall et al., and 125 rad from our calculations).

Regarding the human skeleton (without marrow) as 10% of body mass (19), we calculated that the average skeletal dose from the injection of 1 μCi ^{224}Ra/kg is about 42 rad for children 1-15 years old, 28 rad for adolescents 16-20 years, and 14 rad for adults (8). The corresponding average skeletal dose from the Marshall model would be about 8 rad for adults. Because (a) the Marshall model has not yet been extended to juveniles, and (b) our average skeletal doses are now widely used by clinicians giving ^{224}Ra therapy, and (c) both models will probably require eventual revision, we will continue to use the Spiess and Mays dosimetry until there is solid evidence for change. We prefer one final revision rather than a series of uncertain adjustments.

If Marshall's dosimetry is used, the calculated average skeletal dose would be decreased, and the risk coefficient thereby increased by a factor of 14 rad/8 rad = 1.75 for adults. However, the risk estimate would then be for α-radiation emitted almost entirely from bone surfaces, and this risk estimate for ^{224}Ra might be inappropriately high to apply directly to ^{239}Pu, whose long effective half-life allows time for appreciable burial of the radioactivity within bone volume. A risk reduction factor might then be required which would lower the risk estimate for ^{239}Pu, perhaps to a value similar to that from the Spiess and Mays assumptions.

In effect, our risk estimate for ^{239}Pu assumes that during the tumor induction period, roughly half of the skeletal ^{239}Pu decays on bone surfaces, and half randomly throughout bone volume.

LATENT PERIODS IN MAN

The distribution of appearance times of ^{224}Ra-induced bone sarcomas in 36 of 218 patients injected as juveniles, and in 18 of 682 injected as adults, is shown in Figure 1. For the juveniles at risk, the average year of first injection was 1948 (97% were begun in 1946 through 1951). For the adults at risk in the Spiess series, the average year of first injection was 1951 (2% in 1944-1945, 72% in 1946-1951, 19% in 1952-1957, and 7% in 1958-1964). For all traced patients (alive and dead) the average time of follow-up (from first injection to the last time of known health status) is now 22 years for the juveniles and 19 years for the adults. As of 1976, 33% of the patients injected as juveniles and 43% of the adults are known to have died. For the patients alive in 1976, the average follow-up times are about 28 years for the juveniles and 25 years for the adults.

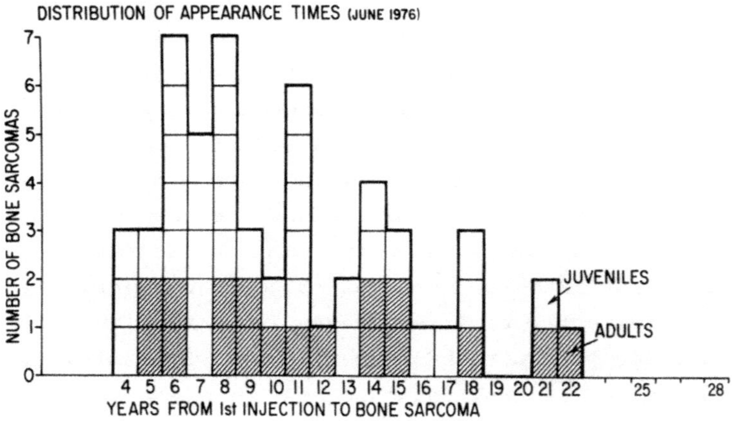

FIGURE 1

Distribution of appearance times of ^{224}Ra-induced bone sarcomas in the Spiess patients. The shortest appearance time was 3 1/2 years (shown rounded to 4 years). The frequency of bone sarcomas peaked at 6 to 8 years and then declined so that after 22 years the risk seems mainly exhausted, especially for those injected as juveniles. Only 1 new bone sarcoma has appeared during the last 6 years. The time from the start of the ^{224}Ra injections to our present 1976 survey averaged 25 years for the adults and 28 years for the juveniles.

As of our present survey in 1976, we have seen no bone sarcomas in patients whose treatments began after 1952, probably due to the lower doses these patients received. Only one new bone sarcoma has appeared since the end of 1969, and that one occurred in an adult in 1972. The present trend suggests that very few additional bone sarcomas are expected to occur among these patients.

The time distribution of ^{224}Ra-induced bone sarcomas is similar to that for leukemias in the A-bomb survivors within 1500 meters of ground zero (20) (Figure 2). The A-bomb irradiation was instantaneous, while that from repeated injections of ^{224}Ra was relatively brief (compared to the long time of follow-up), averaging 6 months for the adults and 11 months for the juveniles. For both leukemia and ^{224}Ra-induced bone sarcomas, the malignancies started to appear within a few years, peaked in frequency at about 6 years, and then declined. The average appearance times of 9 years for leukemia and 10 years for ^{224}Ra-induced bone sarcoma were quite similar. We must emphasize that this similarity pertains to relatively brief irradiation.

In contrast, the appearance times of bone sarcomas induced by continuous irradiation from long-lived ^{226}Ra and ^{228}Ra in humans ranged from 5 to 52 years and averaged 25 years (12). We ascribe these long appearance times to the induction of bone sarcomas by irradiation events received long after

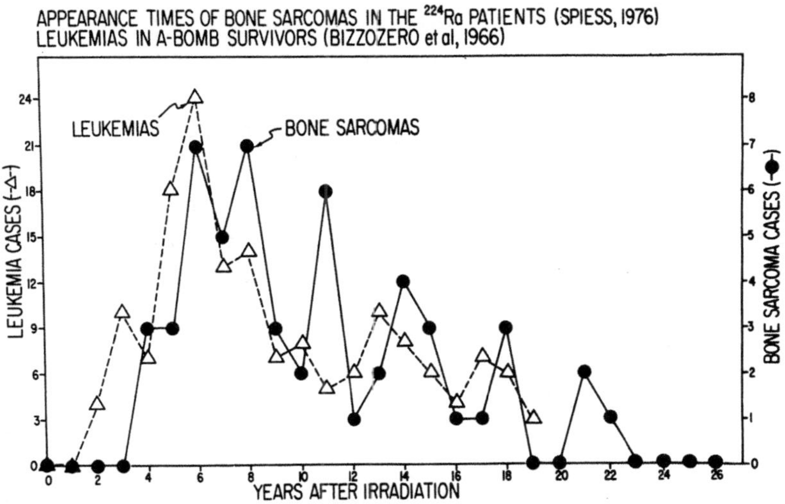

FIGURE 2

Appearance times of bone sarcomas in the ^{224}Ra patients (right ordinate) and leukemias in the A-bomb survivors (left ordinate). The distribution of appearance times is remarkably similar for leukemias (following instantaneous A-bomb irradiation) and for bone sarcomas (following relatively brief ^{224}Ra irradiation).

the start of exposure or, perhaps, the promotion by the delayed irradiation of latent damage received earlier.

PROTRACTION EFFECT

Following a suggestion by Walter A. Müller, we found that for bone sarcoma induction in humans, the effectiveness from a given dose of ^{224}Ra *increased* as the time of irradiation was protracted (9). This effect for ^{224}Ra α-particles, although opposite to that usually observed with sparsely-ionizing X-rays, γ-rays, and β-particles (21), has been confirmed repeatedly in the extensive and well controlled experiments in mice at Neuherberg (5, 22, 23). We have proposed that the observed increase in bone sarcoma incidence for protracted α-particle irradiation from ^{224}Ra might be due to (a) increased number of irradiated cells, (b) less killing of 'premalignant' cells, (c) prolonged stimulus for cell division, and (d) little repair of local damage from α-particles (9, 24).

The exact mathematical expression for the increase in ^{224}Ra effectiveness with protraction is probably quite complicated and may be influenced by many factors, including the size of the dose. However, in the Spiess patients, the observed effectiveness (bone sarcomas per 10^6 person·rad of average skeletal dose) for an injection of x months was well represented by the following simple equations (9):

$$\text{Effectiveness in adults} = 30 + 140\ (1 - e^{-0.09x})$$

$$\text{Effectiveness in juveniles} = 40 + 180\ (1 - e^{-0.09x})$$

For example, the present ^{224}Ra therapy for adult spondylitic patients typically involves 10 injections, totaling 280 μCi ^{224}Ra over a 9 week period (∿ 2 months), for which the calculated average skeletal dose is 56 rad for a 70-kg adult. For this treatment, the computed effectiveness in bone sarcoma production is:

$$30 + 140\ (1 - e^{-(0.09)(2)}) = \frac{53\ \text{bone sarcomas}}{10^6\ \text{person}\cdot\text{rad}}$$

And the calculated risk from this model is:

$$(56\ \text{rad})\left(\frac{53\ \text{bone sarcomas}}{10^6\ \text{person}\cdot\text{rad}}\right) = 0.30\%$$

Using various dose-response models, we have concluded (24) that for the current ^{224}Ra therapy used in Germany, the risk from induced bone sarcoma is small; between 0% (for the threshold model) and 0.5% (for the simple linear model, without a protraction factor). The results of Schales (25) indicate that the actual risk from bone sarcoma is probably within this range for the ^{224}Ra doses now being given to German patients. Thus, unless the risk from other effects, such as kidney disease, liver disease, and cataracts (10) should happen to be appreciable for this treatment, the main factors to consider in the use of ^{224}Ra therapy would be (a) the amount of benefit from the ^{224}Ra treatment, and (b) the availability of alternative modes of therapy with greater benefits, but not appreciably greater risks.

BONE SARCOMA RISK TO MAN

The cumulative risk from ^{224}Ra-induced bone sarcomas, as of our 1976 follow-up, is shown in Figure 3. If the appearance of new bone sarcomas is now essentially exhausted, the observed risk should approximate the life-span risk. A single equation has been used to represent the risk to a population exposed at mixed ages, since juveniles and adults at the same protraction time seem to be at similar risk in terms of calculated average skeletal dose. This equation, which may require future revision, predicts that the number of induced bone sarcomas in 1,000,000 people, each receiving an average skeletal dose of 1 rad from ^{224}Ra (or 10,000 people, each receiving 100 rad, etc.), rises from 40 cases for a single injection of ^{224}Ra, to 200 cases for weekly injections extending over a span of several years.

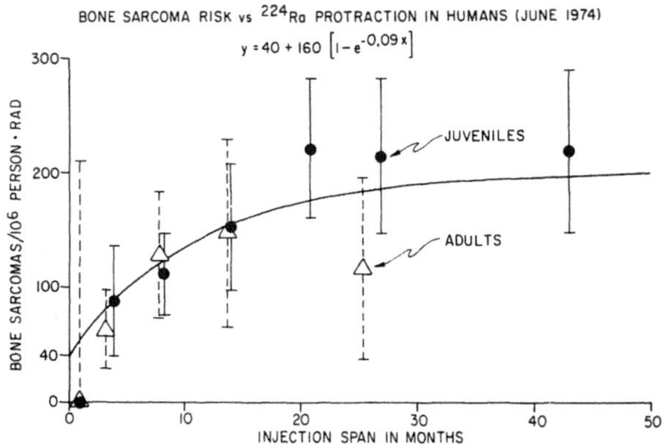

FIGURE 3

Bone sarcoma risk in humans vs. protraction of the ^{224}Ra injections. Data are from the second table of Ref. (9), plus the only additional bone sarcoma known to have occurred in the Spiess patients since the end of 1969 (an adult at 728 rad and 11 months protraction). Standard deviations of each point are shown. The risk rises to about 200 bone sarcomas per 10^6 person·rad for long protraction of irradiation from ^{224}Ra. For a given length of the injections span, and with the dosimetric assumptions that have been used (8), juveniles and adults appear to be roughly similar in bone sarcoma risk per rad from ^{224}Ra.

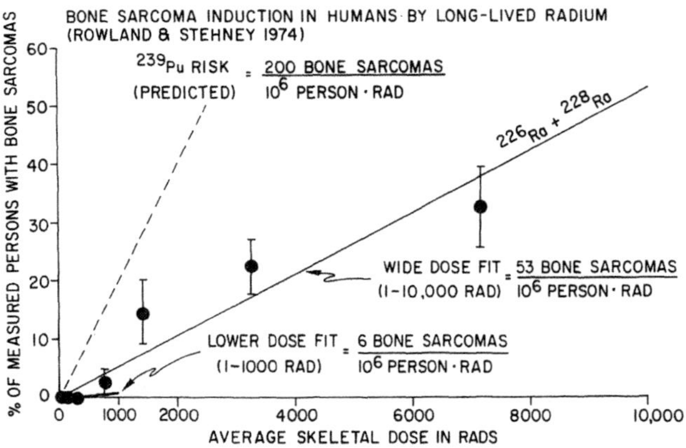

FIGURE 4

Incidence of bone sarcomas in United States persons (mostly dial painters) receiving known skeletal doses from ^{226}Ra and ^{228}Ra (29). Below 10,000 rad, the fitted slope is 53 bone sarcomas/10^6 person·rad. Below 1,000 rad, the fitted slope is 6 bone sarcomas/10^6 person·rad, but this slope is based on only 1 sarcoma case of known dose. If the true risk from low doses of long-lived Radium is between these values, the predicted risk from ^{239}Pu is between 4 and 33 times that from long-lived Radium (15, 16).

^{239}Pu and ^{224}Ra are α-emitters that decay partly on bone surface and partly within bone volume. The limited experimental data in mice and beagles are in accord with the assumption of roughly equal sarcoma risk, per rad of average skeletal dose, for ^{239}Pu and protracted ^{224}Ra (22, 26). Therefore, the risk to the skeleton from lifespan irradiation from ^{239}Pu is taken to be about 200 bone sarcomas/10^6 person·rad. This risk estimate seems correct within a factor of 10 at low doses unless the dose response fails to contain a strong linear component. The upper limit to the risk is established by the lack of bone sarcomas in persons injected with plutonium or exposed to it occupationally (16, 27, 28). The lower limit is established by the fact that the risk per rad of average skeletal dose from ^{239}Pu should be appreciably greater than that from long-lived radium in the United States radium subjects. The risk from bone-surface-seeking ^{239}Pu in animals is 5-20 times that from bone-volume-seeking ^{226}Ra (15, 16).

The data of Rowland and Stehney (29) on the United States dial painters and other persons exposed to long-lived ^{226}Ra and ^{228}Ra are shown in Figure 4. The risk averaged over the wide dose region (0-10,000 rad) was calculated to be 53 bone sarcomas/10^6 person·rad (16), but the risk below 1000 rad could be much lower due to the possibility of a sigmoid dose-response. If the 28 bone sarcoma cases of unknown dose (12) are exhumed and evaluated for retained radium, and if none of their average skeletal doses fall below 1000 rad, this would constitute decisive proof of a decreased risk per rad at low doses of ^{226}Ra in man. Tentatively, the risk below 1000 rad average skeletal dose from ^{226}Ra is taken as between 6 and 53 bone sarcomas/10^6 person·rad. Only one additional case of bone sarcoma has occurred since 1969 among the United States radium subjects, so their bone sarcoma risk seems largely exhausted.

All of the risk estimates in this paper must be regarded as provisional and subject to future revision. The risks from ^{226}Ra-induced carcinomas of the head sinuses, and ^{239}Pu-induced cancers of liver and lung are not included in this paper, but are given in reference (15).

REFERENCES

1. Lloyd, R.D., C.W. Mays, D.R. Atherton and D.O. Clark, The half-period of Ra^{224} (Thorium-X). Research in Radiobiology, University of Utah Report COO-225 (1962) 88-89.
2. Marshall, J.H., The retention of radionuclides in bone. C.W. Mays, W.S.S. Jee, R.D. Lloyd, B.J. Stover, J.H. Dougherty and G.N. Taylor (Ed.): Delayed effects of bone-seeking radionuclides, University of Utah Press, Salt Lake City (1969), 7-27 (particularly, see the comment of R.E. Rowland on page 48 of this book).
3. Marshall, J.H., J. Liniecki, E.L. Lloyd, G. Marotti, C.W. Mays, J. Rundo, H.A. Sissons and W.S. Snyder, Alkaline earth metabolism in adult man. Health Physics 24, 125-221 (1972).
4. Marshall, J.H., P.G. Groer and R.A. Schlenker, Dose to endosteal cells and relative distribution factors for radium-224 and plutonium-239 compared to radium-226. Health Physics (in press).
5. Müller, W.A., W. Gössner, O. Hug and A. Luz, Late effects of short-lived α-emitters. Health Physics (in press).
6. Spiess, H., H. Poppe and H. Schoen, Strahleninduzierte Knochentumoren nach Thorium X-Behandlung. Monatsschrift für Kinderheilkunde 110, 198-201 (1962).
7. Spiess, H., ^{224}Ra-induced tumors in children and adults. C.W. Mays, W.S.S. Jee, R.D. Lloyd, B.J. Stover, J.H. Dougherty and G.N. Taylor (Ed.): Delayed effects of bone-seeking radionuclides, University of Utah Press, Salt Lake City (1969), 227-247.
8. Spiess, H. and C.W. Mays, Bone cancers induced by ^{224}Ra (ThX) in children and adults. Health Physics 19, 713-729 (1970), plus addendum, Health Physics 20, 543-545 (1971).
9. Spiess, H. and C.W. Mays, Protraction effect on bone sarcoma induction of ^{224}Ra in children and adults.

In: C.L. Sanders, R.H. Busch, J.E. Ballou and D.D. Mahlum (Ed.), Radionuclide carcinogenesis, AEC Symposium Series 29, CONF-720505 (1973), 437-450.

10. Spiess, H., A. Gerspach and C.W. Mays, Soft-tissue effects following ^{224}Ra injections into humans. Health Physics (in press).

11. Mays, C.W., H. Spiess and A. Gerspach, Skeletal effects following ^{224}Ra injections into humans. Health Physics (in press).

12. Keane, A.T., A.F. Stehney and R.E. Rawland, Appearance times of human bone tumors induced by skeletal deposits of radium. Radiat.Res. 67, 625-626 (1976).

13. Jee, W.S.S., J.S. Arnold, T.H. Cochran, J.A. Twente and R.S. Mical, Relationship of microdistribution of alpha particles to damage. T.F. Dougherty, W.S.S. Jee, C.W. Mays and B.J. Stover (Ed.): Some aspects of internal irradiation, Pergamon Press, Oxford (1962), 27-45.

14. Jee, W.S.S., B.J. Stover, G.N. Taylor and W.R. Christensen, The skeletal toxicity of Pu^{239} in adult beagles. Health Physics 8, 599-607 (1962).

15. Mays, C.W., Estimated risk from ^{239}Pu to human bone, liver, and lung. M. Lewis (Ed.): Biological and environmental effects of low level radiation, Vol. II, IAEA, Vienna (1976), 373-384.

16. Mays, C.W., H. Spiess, G.N. Taylor, R.D. Lloyd, W.S.S. Jee, S. McFarland, D.H. Taysum, T.W. Brammer, D. Brammer and T.A. Pollard, Estimated risk to human bone from ^{239}Pu. W.S.S. Jee (Ed.): The health effects of plutonium and radium, J.W. Press, Anatomy Dept., University of Utah, Salt Lake City (1976), 343-362.

17. Barr, N.F. and E. Sinclair, Personal communication to C.W. Mays (August 1976).

18. Maletskos, C.J., A.T. Keane, N.C. Telles and R.D. Evans, Retention and absorption of ^{224}Ra and ^{234}Th and some dosimetric consequences of ^{224}Ra in human beings. C.W. Mays, W.S.S. Jee, R.D. Lloyd, B.J. Stover, J.H. Dougherty and G.N. Taylor (Ed.): Delayed effects

of bone-seeking radionuclides, University of Utah Press, Salt Lake City (1969), 29-49.

19. Snyder, W.S., M.J. Cook, L.R. Karhausen, E.S. Nasset, G.P. Howells,and I.H. Tipton, Report of the task group on reference man, ICRP report 23, Pergamon Press, Oxford (1975), 290-291.

20. Bizzozero, O.J., K.G. Johnson and A. Ciocco, Radiation-related leukemia in Hiroshima and Nagasaki 1946-1964. New England J.Med. 274, 1095-1101 (1966).

21. Mays, C.W., R.D. Lloyd and J.H. Marshall, Malignancy risk to humans from total body γ-ray irradiation. W.S. Snyder (Ed.): Proceedings of the third international congress of the international radiation protection association, USAEC CONF-730907, U.S. National Technical Information Service, Springfield, Virginia (1974), 417-428.

22. Erfle, V., W. Gössner, O. Hug, A. Luz, K.H. Marquart and W.A. Müller, Reports on the Neuherberg long-term experiments with short-lived alpha emitters (Part 1): The dependence of late effects in mice on the temporal distribution of skeletal alpha-doses from Ra-224 and Th-227. (This symposium).

23. Luz, A., W.A. Müller, W. Gössner and O. Hug, Estimation of tumour risk at low dose from experimental results after incorporation of short-lived bone-seeking alpha emitters ^{224}Ra and ^{227}Th in mice. M. Lewis (Ed.): Biological and environmental effects of low-level radiation, Vol. II, IAEA, Vienna (1976), 171-181.

24. Mays, C.W., Cancer induction in man from internal radioactivity. Health Physics 25, 585-592 (1973).

25. Schales, F., Problems and results of a new follow-up study: ^{224}Ra in adult ankylosing spondylitis patients. (This symposium).

26. Mays, C.W., R.D. Lloyd, G.N. Taylor and D.R. Atherton, Ra toxicity from a pilot study in beagles. Research in Radiobiology, University of Utah Report COO-119-252 (March 1977). (Preprints available from C.W. Mays).

27. Rowland, R.E. and P.W. Durbin, Survival, causes of death

and estimated tissue doses in a group of human beings injected with plutonium. W.S.S. Jee (Ed.): The health effects of plutonium and radium, J.W. Press, University of Utah, Salt Lake City (1976), 329-341.

28. Hempelmann, L.H., W.H. Langham, C.R. Richmond and G. Voelz, Manhattan project plutonium workers: A 27-year follow up study of selected cases. Health Physics 25, 461-479 (1973).

29. Rowland, R.E. and A.F. Stehney, Exposure data for radium patients. Argonne National Laboratory Report ANL-75-3, Part II (1974), 177-231.

Problems in radiological protection involving α-emitters in bone

G.W. Dolphin

National Radiological Protection Board
Harwell, Didcot, Oxon OX11 ORQ, UK

ABSTRACT

Quantitative dose-effect relationships for humans exposed to α-emitters can only be established from data on humans exposed to this type of radiation. The risk of bone sarcoma from exposure to ^{239}Pu may be established from the data on the human cases exposed to ^{226}Ra either by consideration of the radiation dose to the osteoprogenitor cells or by use of the average bone dose together with a modifying factor to take into account the greater toxicity of plutonium relative to radium. The relative toxicity can be evaluated from the data on osteosarcoma incidence in animals. Both methods of risk estimation are given and criticised in the paper.

In future recommendations, ICRP will not use the critical organ concept and the late effects from α-emitters deposited in organs other than the bone will have to be taken into account in setting maximum permissible annual intakes. The implications of this and other proposed changes in ICRP concepts are discussed.

INTRODUCTION

Over the last few years the attention of the public has been drawn both to the limitations of world energy supplies and to their increasing rate of use. Known oil and gas reserves are expected to be exhausted in about 100 years and coal reserves in a few hundred years. Nuclear fission of ^{235}U in thermal reactors is beginning to supply a modest fraction of the total energy requirements of the developed countries. However, supplies of ^{235}U are far from plentiful and it is predicted that they will be exhausted within about 100 years. The long-term future of nuclear fission requires the use of fast reactor systems to produce ^{239}Pu from ^{238}U, which is 140 times more abundant than ^{235}U. Hence the production and use of plutonium is an integral part of the future supplies of energy from nuclear fission reactors. The other α-emitting higher actinides, americium and curium, will be associated with plutonium in these reactors.

For many different reasons groups of scientists and informed laymen have objected to nuclear reactors as a source of energy. Part of their argument has been on radiological protection grounds in that plutonium and the higher actinides produced in thermal fission reactors and used as fuel in fast breeder reactors are very dangerous materials. A frequently quoted example is that a few kilograms, a sphere about the size of an orange, would eventually induce cancers in the whole population of the United Kingdom, provided that the plutonium could be distributed equally among the 55 million inhabitants. Tamplin and Cochran (1974) have claimed that the present allowable level in lung, 0.016 μCi of ^{239}Pu which delivers a dose at a rate of 15 rem per year, is about 115,000 times too high when related to 'hot' particles of plutonium dioxide. In later publications this claim was reduced to 1,000. More recently Morgan (1975) in a paper which has been heavily criticised by the author and many other scientists suggested that the current maximum permissible body burden (MPBB) for ^{239}Pu was about 240 times too high.

The purpose of this paper is to review some of the problems in radiological protection associated with α-emitters in bone. Mays et al. (1976), Mays (1976) and Dolphin et al. (1974) have reviewed this subject in detail so that little fresh can be added but this paper may serve a useful purpose by reaching a different audience and a wider range of readers.

HUMAN RADIUM CASES

Quantitative data on the risks of cancer in irradiated humans can only be obtained from epidemiological studies of human populations. Furthermore human data on the risks from high LET radiation cannot be derived with any certainty from estimated risks of low LET radiation using the conventional dosimetric models and RBE values because the spatial and temporal deposition of energy in tissues by α-particles and γ-radiation are very different. Also, the effects of oxygen and dose rate on the biological damage caused by low and high LET radiation vary considerably. Hence the starting point for assessing quantitatively the biological effects of α-emitters in bone must be the human cases contaminated with radium in the first half of this century.

Data on the human experience of internal contamination with ^{226}Ra in the USA have been collected at the Center for Human Radiobiology and the latest data available on the average doses to bone in 1740 cases are given in ANL 75-60 (1975) and are shown in Table I. For a linear dose-effect

TABLE I

THE DISTRIBUTION OF 1740 RADIUM CASES INCLUDING THOSE WITH SARCOMAS AND CANCERS OF THE EPITHELIAL TISSUE ADJACENT TO BONE SURFACES IN ARBITRARILY CHOSEN RANGES OF AVERAGE DOSE TO BONE (ANL 75-60, 1975)

	Average dose to bone (rads)					
	0	1-300	-1000	-3000	-10000	>10000
Cases	389	1063	83	74	90	41
Sarcomas	-	-	1	14	24	15
Cancers	-	-	1	6	15	5
Population dose	-	41727	46608	138141	499784	734328

Risk 53 sarcomas/10^6 man-rads

Risk 30 cancers/10^6 man-rads

relationship the risk of bone sarcoma is $53/10^6$ man-rads and for cancer of the epithelial tissues adjacent to bone $30/10^6$ man-rads. In this analysis cases with an average dose to bone above 10,000 rads have been neglected as they appear to have a considerably lower risk which could be due to an over-kill effect. As will be noted later, the risk of bone sarcoma for humans based on the average dose to bone is six times less than that for beagles which illustrates the uncertainty in extrapolating risk data from one species to another.

There are well recognised problems with these human data which are related to the manner in which data on the cases have been collected. Some cases have been included because they came to notice as a result of clinical symptoms which may have biased the risk estimate upwards. On the other hand not all the cases have died so that a few more bone sarcomas may yet occur (Rowland, 1975).

The value of 0.1 μCi of ^{226}Ra has been recommended by the International Commission on Radiological Protection (ICRP) as the MPBB for over 20 years and it was based on an assessment of the earlier data available from the radium cases. If this MPBB were maintained in the bone for 50 years it would give an accumulated average dose to bone of about 200 rads which corresponds to a risk of just over 1.5% of a sarcoma plus cancer. However, the ICRP recommendations refer to a uniform accumulation resulting in an MPBB at the end of a working life of 50 years. This chronic accumulation of radium leads to a lower total dose and the associated risk would be less than 1%.

The evaluation of the risk of a malignancy has been based on the average dose to bone. In 1967 a report was prepared for ICRP (ICRP, 1968) in which the cells at risk in bone were identified as osteoprogenitors, lining bone surfaces, particularly the endosteal surfaces. It is from these cells that osteosarcomas appear to originate. This publication by ICRP stimulated many workers, particularly Spiers and his group at Leeds, Beddoe et al. (1976), Harley and Pasternak (1976) and Thorne (1976) to make measurements and estimates of doses to osteoprogenitor cells and bone marrow cells. The calculated doses to the osteoprogenitor cells, D_{op}, are frequently expressed in terms of the average dose to bone, D_{av}. For ^{226}Ra, on the assumption that 30% of radon and daughter products are retained in the bone, the average dose rate is:

$$D_{av} = 51.2 \times \frac{I}{5000} \times 10.9 \text{ rads/day}$$

where 51.2 is the well-known constant;
I is the content in μCi;
5000 g is the mass of mineral bone (ICRP, 1975); and
10.9 MeV is the energy deposited in bone/disintegration of ^{226}Ra.

The dose rate to the osteoprogenitor cells from a bone content of I μCi may be calculated on the assumption that the sensitive volume, the cell nucleus, is at an average distance of 10 μm from the bone surface. As the dose rate from α-emitters in bone falls rapidly with distance, the location of the cells relative to the surface is important. However, for purposes of comparison of the dose rate from ^{226}Ra with that from ^{239}Pu, within limits, this distance may not be quite so critical. Harley and Pasternak (1976) have calculated doses from ^{226}Ra in bone at various distances from bone surfaces and from their results:

$$D_{op} = \frac{I}{2500} \times 103.6 \text{ rads/day}$$

where $\frac{I}{2500}$ μCi/cm³ is the bone content per unit volume assuming a bone density of 2 g/cm³; and
103.6 rads/day at 10 μm from the bone surface per μCi/cm³ is taken from Harley and Pasternak (1976) but adjusted for 30% retention of radon and daughters.

Hence $$D_{op} = \frac{D_{av} \times \frac{I}{2500} \times 103.6}{51.2 \times \frac{I}{5000} \times 10.9} = 0.37\ D_{av}$$

This relationship may be used to express the risk of sarcoma and cancer in terms of the dose to the osteoprogenitor cells as 143 and 81 per 10^6 man-rads respectively. These values of risk are higher than those obtained using the average dose to bone indicating that risk values depend on the choice of the dosimetric model.

ESTIMATION OF MPBB FOR PLUTONIUM FROM DATA ON THE RADIUM CASES

If the assumption that bone sarcomas arise from the osteoprogenitor cells and that the risk of sarcoma is linearly proportional to the α-radiation dose is correct, then the amount of ^{239}Pu in the bones, biologically equivalent to 0.1 μCi of ^{226}Ra, can be calculated. However, there are many problems with this approach arising from the differences in metabolism between radium and plutonium.

Radium taken into the body over a long period, as in occupational exposures, will become uniformly distributed throughout the bone with perhaps a few 'hot' spots in those regions where bone deposition was taking place at times when the radium concentration in the plasma was high (Rowland, 1960). The natural processes of resorption and deposition continue throughout life and these tend to increase the uniformity of the distribution of radium in mineral bone.

Plutonium enters the body through the lungs or a wound site and is transported in the blood and body fluids mainly bound to transferrin, the molecule involved in iron transport. A small fraction is bound to citrate. At bone surfaces the plutonium is exchanged on to other binding sites which appear to be associated with mucoproteins in the non-mineralised component of bone (Chipperfield and Taylor, 1972). With time the surface deposits become buried or removed by the resorption and deposition processes. The rate of removal from bone surfaces has not been established with certainty in animals and furthermore in many experiments with animals relatively large amounts of plutonium have been used and the radiation dose could have affected the natural processes involved in resorption and deposition. An interesting new experimental technique has been developed by Priest (1977) who showed by autoradiographic methods that in hamsters and rats the soft β-emitting isotope, ^{241}Pu injected as citrate, rapidly appears inside cells on bone surfaces, initially in the nucleus and later in the cytoplasm. This observation may affect present views about the location of plutonium in bone surfaces as expressed above. In studies of the micro-distribution near vertebral bone surfaces in rats injected with plutonium citrate, Storr et al. (1975) showed that more than half the plutonium was near the surface on day one but after a year more than half the plutonium was beyond 15 μm from the surface. This movement of the plutonium would lower the dose rate at 10 μm from the surface by more than 50%. As yet there are no data available on the movement of plutionium from bone surfaces in man but some are expected from current studies at the Center for Human Radiobiology.

The relationship between the average dose to bone and the dose to the osteoprogenitor cells may be calculated for ^{239}Pu from the data given by Harley and Pasternak (1976):

$$D_{av} = 51.2 \times \frac{I}{5000} \times 5.51 \text{ rads/day}$$

where 5.15 MeV is the energy per disintegration of ^{239}Pu.

$$D_{op} = \frac{I}{120{,}000} \times 46.8 \times 10^3$$

where 120,000 cm^2 is the surface area of bone on which the plutonium is assumed to be uniformly deposited in a one micron thick layer; and

46.8 x 10^3 rads/day is the dose rate at 10 μm from bone surfaces per $\mu Ci/cm^2$.

Hence $D_{op} = 7.4\ D_{av}$

With the passage of time after deposition in bone there is a gradual change to a more uniform distribution of the plutonium throughout the bone. For example, if the plutonium is uniformly mixed in a 24 μm layer of bone surface then the dose rate at 10 μm from the bone surface is reduced to 18.7×10^3 rads/day for an initial deposit of 1 $\mu Ci/cm^2$. However, if the plutonium becomes uniformly mixed in trabecular bone this dose rate is reduced further to 5.38×10^3 rads/day.

Hence $D_{op} = D_{av} \times 3.0$

for mixing in a 24 μm layer according to the data given by Harley and Pasternak (1976); and

$D_{op} = D_{av} \times 0.85$

for uniform mixing in trabecular bone.

The effect of these two dosimetry models and the three selected distributions of the plutonium on the estimated risk of bone sarcoma from ^{226}Ra and ^{239}Pu, and the bone content of ^{239}Pu which is equivalent to 0.1 μCi of ^{226}, are summarised in Table II. In this table it is assumed that for equal risks

TABLE II

RISK OF BONE SARCOMAS IN HUMANS CALCULATED FOR EXPOSURE TO PLUTONIUM-239 FROM DATA ON RADIUM-226 CASES USING TWO DOSIMETRIC MODELS. THE BONE CONTENT OF PLUTONIUM-239 EQUIVALENT TO 0.1 Ci OF RADIUM-226 IS ALSO GIVEN

Dosimetric model	Risk of sarcoma from ^{226}Ra x 10^6 man-rads	Plutonium-239 Assumed distribution in bone	Plutonium-239 Risk of sarcoma x 10^6 man-rads	Bone content of ^{239}Pu equivalent to 0.1 μCi ^{226}Ra (μCi)
Average dose to bone	53	in 1 μm layer	1060	0.01
		in 24 μm layer	420	0.03
		uniform**	120	0.09
Dose to osteoprogenitor cells at 10 μm from surface	143	in 1 μm layer	143*	0.01
		in 24 μm layer	143*	0.03
		uniform**	143*	0.09

* Assumed risks equal to that for ^{226}Ra

** Surface deposit on trabecular bone uniformly mixed in trabecular bone

of sarcoma from ^{226}Ra and ^{239}Pu the doses delivered to the osteoprogenitor cells from these radionuclides should be the same. Hence the risk of sarcoma estimated for the average dose model is obtained using the relationship between D_{op} and D_{av} given above.

The risk estimates given in the table for ^{239}Pu in the bone range from 120 to 1060 sarcomas/10^6 man-rads. This large range clearly shows how the estimated risk depends on the dosimetric model and the assumed distribution of plutonium in the bone. The amount of ^{239}Pu in the bone equivalent to 0.1 μCi of ^{226}Ra given in the last column of the table has a range which includes the value of 0.04 μCi currently recommended for the whole body by ICRP (1959).

There is not sufficient information on plutonium metabolism in bone to allow the most appropriate model for distribution to be chosen. Mays et al. (1976) have suggested a model whereby half the dose is delivered from surface deposits of plutonium and the other half from a uniform distribution; this represents the two extremes of distribution. For this model an average risk would be about 500 per 10^6 man-rads corresponding to ^{239}Pu being about ten times more toxic than ^{226}Ra. However, there is no biological evidence to support this model. The present indications are that ICRP dose calculations will be based on a surface distribution of plutonium with a retention half-life of 100 years. This is obviously a very conservative model.

^{224}RA IN HUMANS

The biological effects caused by the injection of ^{224}Ra into humans for the treatment of tuberculosis and ankylosing spondylitis have been reviewed by Spiess and Mays (1970 and 1973) and summarised by Mays et al. (1976). The interpretation of these very interesting biological data in terms of dose-effect relationships is hampered by the lack of an agreed dosimetric model. A fraction of the injected activity will decay on bone surfaces, and another fraction in the bone volume; some of the activity will decay in the body fluids before deposition in bone can occur. Although it has been suggested that ^{224}Ra may be an analogue for ^{239}Pu, in respect of its radiocarcinogenic properties as both are assumed to decay on bone surfaces, this suggestion is altogether too simplistic to merit serious consideration.

RELATIVE TOXICITY OF ^{226}RA AND ^{239}PU IN BEAGLES

In the previous section a range of bone contents for plutonium was derived from human data on the radium cases. Here it is proposed to review the relevant data on beagles exposed by intravenous injection at the University of Utah which have been reported in detail in the Annual Reports of the Radiobiology Division (1975). From the initial experiments which were completed some years ago, data from four groups of dogs injected with ^{226}Ra and three groups injected with ^{239}Pu can be used to obtain risk values for these animals.

For the dogs exposed to ^{226}Ra the retentions were measured in individual dogs and the average dose to bone calculated for each group. In the groups listed in Table III the average radon retention in the bones was 25% (Lloyd, 1970). The average dose to bone was calculated by Mays et al. (1976) up to one year before death when the malignancy was assumed to have been initiated. The dose to the osteoprogenitor cells at 10 μm from the bone surface, D_{op}, may be estimated from the average dose to bone, D_{av}, for beagles using the data given by Harley and Pasternak (1976).

$$D_{av} = 51.2 \times \frac{I}{640} \times 9.9 \text{ rads/day}$$

where 640 g is the mass of the mineral bone in beagles;
9.9 MeV is the energy/disintegration of ^{226}Ra adjusted for 25% retention of radon: and

$$D_{op} = \frac{I}{320} \times 86.3 \text{ rads/day}$$

where 320 cm^3 is the bone volume with a density of 2 g/cm^3; 86.3 rads/day for a bone content of 1 $\mu Ci/cm$.

Therefore $D_{op} = 0.34\ D_{av}$

and this relationship is used to calculate the doses to the osteoprogenitor cells in the dogs injected with ^{226}Ra in Table III.

TABLE III

SKELETAL RADIATION DOSE CALCULATED USING TWO DOSIMETRIC MODELS AND BONE SARCOMA IN BEAGLES INJECTED WITH RADIUM-226 AND PLUTONIUM-239 AT THE UNIVERSITY OF UTAH

Nuclide	Injected amount µCi/kg	Years to death	Sarcomas / dogs	Average dose to 1 yr before death: Bone D_{av} rads	Average dose to 1 yr before death: Cells* D_{op} rads	Dose for 1% incidence: Bone rads	Dose for 1% incidence: Cells* rads
^{226}Ra	0.058	11.2	0/12	183	62	-	-
	0.166	9.40	1/14	447	151	64	7.2
	0.339	10.05	5/13	1100	374	29	9.8
	1.07	6.12	11/12	2500	850	27	9.2
^{239}Pu	0.016	10.54	4/14	55	297	1.9	10.2
	0.048	8.22	10/14	135	729	1.9	10.3
	0.095	6.83	10/12	231	1247	2.8	15

* Osteoprogenitor cells 10 µm from bone surface

The average dose to bone for the dogs injected with plutonium was calculated for the individual dogs using the retention equation for bone following an injection of unit activity:

$$R = 0.286e^{-0.0011t} + 0.21$$

where t is in days (Stover, 1976) and the values given in Table III are taken from Mays et al. (1976).

Again, the relationship between the average dose to bone and the dose to the osteoprogenitor cells from plutonium on the surface was obtained from data taken from Harley and Pasternak (1976) and is:

$$D_{op} = 5.4\ D_{av}$$

This relationship is slightly different from that derived for humans due to differences in the surface to volume ratio in the two species. This relationship is used to derive the dose given in column 6 of Table III for ^{239}Pu. It is noted that the doses to the osteoprogenitor cells are higher than the average dose to bone and this appears to make the radionuclide less effective in producing sarcomas. This apparent effect is due to the assumption that all the plutonium is located on bone surfaces. As in the previous section, two other examples of plutonium distribution are considered. For distribution in a layer 24 μm thick in the bone surface:

$$D_{op} = 2.2\ D_{av}$$

and for uniform mixing in trabecular bone:

$$D_{op} = 0.62\ D_{av}$$

The risks of bone sarcoma from ^{226}Ra and ^{239}Pu calculated for two different dosimetric models and three different distributions of plutonium are given in Table IV and they range over a factor of 15. The relative toxicity is given in the third line of the table and the value of 0.9 could indicate that the dose to the osteoprogenitors with a surface distribution is the most appropriate one to calculate for it gives roughly equal toxicities. However, this calculation is based on the unrealistic assumption that there is no burial or removal of plutonium from bone surfaces.

In the last line of the table the bone content of ^{239}Pu equivalent to 0.1 μCi of ^{226}Ra in bone of humans is given for the relevant toxicity values. These bone contents are in the same range as those in Table II, 0.01-0.1 μCi, which includes 0.04 μCi.

TABLE IV

RISK OF BONE SARCOMA IN BEAGLES CALCULATED FOR TWO DIFFERENT DOSIMETRIC MODELS AND FOR THREE DISTRIBUTIONS OF PLUTONIUM IN BONE SURFACE

	Risk of bone sarcoma x 10^6 beagle-rads for two dosimetric models			
	Average dose to bone	Dose to osteoprogenitor cells at 10 μm from the surface		
		Surface distribution	Mixed in 24 μm layer	Uniform distribution*
^{226}Ra	320	-	-	940
^{239}Pu	4420	820	2000	6900
Relative toxicity	14	0.9	2	7
Body content (μCi) of ^{239}Pu in humans corresponding to 0.1 μCi of ^{226}Ra	0.012	0.012	0.029	0.10

* Surface deposit on trabecular bone uniformly mixed trabecular bone

EXPERIENCE WITH PLUTONIUM IN HUMANS

Few details have been published on the health experience and causes of death of workers exposed to plutonium. Hempelmann et al. (1973) reported on the health of 25 males who were exposed to plutonium 27 years previously. Body contents in these men, estimated by urinary excretion analysis, ranged from 5 to 420 μCi but these estimates could be too high for it is known that urinary excretion methods often over-estimate body content. No abnormal health problems have been seen in these men. Voelz (1975) has given information about occupational plutonium exposures in the USA and recorded 28 workers with body contents estimated to be over 0.04 μCi. In the United Kingdom Schofield (1976) reported 14 workers at BNFL Windscale, with body contents over 0.04 μCi. No bone sarcomas or any excess of other cancers attributable to the plutonium exposure have been reported in these groups or in other persons occupationally exposed to plutonium.

The most relevant experience of plutonium in the body comes from the data given by Rowland and Durbin (1976) on 18 people who were injected with plutonium in the USA in 1944-1945. These cases are estimated to have accumulated a dose to bone of 1050 man-rads. Although some survived only a few months, 8 survived for at least 8 years and 4 were still alive in 1975. No bone sarcomas or other malignancies which could be attributed to plutonium have been reported.

Although the human experience with plutonium is limited it is sufficient to rule out excessive claims about its toxicity. However, looking to the future the most reliable evidence on the toxicity of plutonium will come from the extensive study of human experience. In the United Kingdom a Registry for Radiation Workers is being set up which will include details of the estimated body content of plutonium as well as the external radiation dose. These radiation dose records will be associated eventually with the cause of death so that the age specific death rate of workers exposed to plutonium may be compared with those of other workers who have not been exposed (Reissland et al., 1976).

RADIOLOGICAL PROTECTION ASPECTS

In ICRP Publication 2 (1959) values for MPC_a, MPC_w and MPBB were calculated from the basic radiation dose standards of 5, 15 or 30 rem in a year to the whole body or a critical organ. The single critical organ concept used in this publication is now losing favour in the development of new ICRP recommendations. The main disadvantage of this concept is that it does not take into account that several organs may be irradiated to a significant level following an intake. For example, inhaled plutonium delivers a significant dose to the lung, liver and bone. Hence there is a risk of late effects developing in all three organs not just in the critical organ receiving the highest dose. In its new formulations Committee 2 of ICRP will add the risks to the three organs in this particular case and the annual limit on intake will be based on the total risk from the three organs. Now it will become important to quantify the risk from α-irradiation of other organs, such as lung and liver, as well as to the bone. The main disadvantage of this system is that it requires a more exact knowledge of the risks of cancer in individual organs than is available at present. It also makes the assumption that the risk to the whole body is the sum of the risks to the individual organs which is not necessarily correct. If there are immunological factors involved in the development of cancer then the integral dose and total mass of tissue irradiated may be important factors.

The other major development in radiological protection is that the average dose to bone model is being discarded in favour of the calculation of dose to the osteoprogenitor cells on bone surfaces. Most of the advantages and disadvantages of this dosimetric model have already been mentioned in this paper. For radiological protection purposes the main advantage is that a uniform system of dosimetry can be used for both α- and β-emitters in the bone. The main disadvantage is that it is a complex model which cannot be accommodated within the bounds of our present poor knowledge of bone structure, bone turnover kinetics and location of the sites of deposition for those elements associated with the non-mineral component of bone. Also the use of this model involves assumptions about uniformity of deposition on bone surfaces, uniformity of distribution of osteo-rog progenitor cells on these surfaces and concentrates entirely on endosteal surfaces excluding surfaces in Haversian canals and surfaces of the periosteum. The adoption of doses to osteoprogenitor cells as the basis for radiological protection recommendations is not convincing at the moment due to the lack of detailed knowledge.

FUTURE DEVELOPMENTS

Most of the future developments required for radiological

protection purposes have already been discussed and they include more data on:

a. health and causes of death of workers exposed to α-emitting radionuclides;
b. the relative biological effects in large experimental animals for at present there are data on only 17 sarcomas in 51 beagles caused by ^{226}Ra and 24 sarcomas in 40 beagles injected with ^{239}Pu at the University of Utah;
c. bone structure and remodelling rates including surface to volume ratio and its variation among bones in the skeleton;
d. cell localisation and kinetics on bone surfaces;
e. sites of deposition and retention of plutonium and higher actinides in bone. The recent work of Priest (1976) has cast doubt on the conventional views about plutonium bound to mucoproteins in non-mineral bone and emphasises the role of the bone cells in plutonium metabolism.

ACKNOWLEDGEMENTS

The author wishes to thank Mrs Elaine Henry for her help with the manuscript.

REFERENCES

1. Argonne National Laboratory, Radiological and Environmental Research Division Annual Report. ANL-75-60 Part II. Center for Human Radiobiology, Argonne (1975).
2. Beddoe, H.A., P.J. Darley and F.W. Spiers, Measurements of trabecular bone structure in man. Phys.Med.Biol. 21, 589 (1976).
3. Chipperfield, A.R. and D.M. Taylor, The binding of thorium (IV), plutonium (IV), americium (III) and curium (III) to the constituents of bovine cortical bone *in vitro*. Radiation Res. 51, 15 (1972).
4. Dolphin, G.W., H. Smith, D.S. Popplewell, J.W. Stather, N, Adams, N.L. Spoor, J. Brightwell and R.A. Bulman,

Radiological problems in the protection of persons exposed to plutonium. National Radiological Protection Board Report No. R-29 (1974).

5. Harley, N.H. and B.S. Pasternak, A comparison of the dose to cells on trabecular bone surfaces from ^{239}Pu and ^{226}Ra based on experimental α absorption measurements. Health Physics 30, 35 (1976).
6. Hempelmann, L.H., W.H. Langham, C.R. Richmond and G.L. Voelz, Manhattan Project Plutonium Workers: A 27-year follow-up study of selected cases. Health Physics 25, 461 (1973).
7. International Commission on Radiological Protection, Permissible doses for internal radiation. ICRP Publication 2. Pergamon Press, Oxford 1959.
8. International Commission on Radiological Protection, A review of the radiosensitivity of tissues in bone. ICRP Publication 11. Pergamon Press, Oxford 1968.
9. International Commission on Radiological Protection, Report of the Task Group on Reference Man. ICRP Publication 23. Pergamon Press, Oxford 1975.
10. Lloyd, R.D., Retention and dosimetry of some injected radionuclides in beagles. University of Utah Report COO-119-241 (1970).
11. Mays, C.W., Estimated risk from plutonium-239 to human bone, liver and lung. Proc.Symp.Biological Effects of Low Level Radiation, IAEA, Vienna 1976.
12. Mays, C.W., H. Spiess, G.N. Taylor, R.D. Lloyd, W.S.S. Jee, S. McFarland, D.H. Taysum, T.W. Brammer, D. Brammer and T.A. Pollard, Estimated risk to human bone from plutonium-239. Health Effects of Plutonium and Radium. W.S.S. Jee (Ed.), J.W. Press, University of Utah (1976).
13. Morgan, K.Z., Suggested reduction of permissible exposure to plutonium and other transuranic elements. Amer. industr.Hyg.Assoc.J. 36, 565 (1975).
14. Priest, N., The distribution of plutonium-241 in rodents. Int.J.Radiat.Biol. 31, 59 (1977).
15. Reissland, J.A., P. Kay and G.W. Dolphin, The observation and analysis of cancer deaths among classified radi-

ation workers. Phys.Med.Biol. 21, 903 (1976).

16. Rowland, R.E., Radioisotopes in the skeleton: late observations on the distribution of radium in the human skeleton. p. 339 In: A Symposium on Radioisotopes in the Biosphere. R.S. Caldecott and L.A. Snyder (Eds.), University of Minnesota (1960).

17. Rowland, R.E., The risk of malignancy from internally deposited radioisotopes. p. 146 In: Proc. 5th Intern. Congr. Radiation Res. O.F. Nygaards, H.I. Adler and W.K. Sinclair (Eds.), Academic Press, N.Y. 1975.

18. Rowland, R.E. and P.W. Durbin, Survival, causes of death and estimated tissue doses in a group of human beings injected with plutonium. p. 329 In: The Health Effects of Plutonium and Radium. W.S.S. Jee (Ed.), J.W. Press, University of Utah (1976).

19. Schofield, G.B. Personal communication (1976).

20. Spiess, H. and C.W. Mays, Bone cancers induced by radium-224 in children and adults. Health Physics 19, 713 (1970).

21. Spiess, H. and C.W. Mays, Protraction effect on bone sarcoma induction of radium-224 in children and adults. p. 437 In: Radionuclide Carcinogenesis. C.L. Sanders, R.H. Busch, J.E. Ballou and D.D. Mahlum (Eds.). US Atomic Energy Commission, Washington 1973.

22. Storr, M.C., J.G. Hollings and R.L. Clarke, An improved method of fission fragment radiography of plutonium in rat bone. Intern.J.appl. Radiation & Isotopes 26, 708 (1975).

23. Stover, B.J., Skeletal dosimetry in the beagle. p. 97 In: Health Effects of Plutonium and Radium. W.S.S. Jee (Ed.), J.W. Press, University of Utah (1976).

24. Tamplin, A.R. and T.B. Cochran, Radiation standards for hot particles: A report on the inadequacy of existing radiological standards related to internal exposure of man. National Resources Defense Council, Washington 1974.

25. Thorne, M.C., Aspects of the dosimetry of plutonium in bone. Nature 259, 539 (1976).

26. University of Utah, Research in Radiobiology. Annual Report of Work in Progress in the Internal Irradiation Program. COO-119-250 (1975).
27. Voelz, G.L., What we have learned about plutonium from human data. Health Physics 29, 551 (1975).

A model for the induction of bone cancer by ^{224}Ra*

P.G. Groer and J.H. Marshall

Radiological and Environmental Research Division
Argonne National Laboratory, 9700 South Cass Avenue,
Argonne, Illinois 60439

ABSTRACT

A mathematical model for the transformation of normal endosteal cells into malignant tumor cells by α-irradiation is applied to ^{224}Ra. The model postulates that a normal endosteal cell near the bone surface is transformed into a malignant cell by three consecutive events. The first two events are the initiation events. The probability of their occurrence is proportional to the absorbed endosteal dose and they generate dormant tumor cells. These dormant tumor cells are promoted by the third event, the promotion event. The probability of this last event is proportional to the rate of bone remodeling but independent of the radiation dose. In competition with these transforming events is the killing of any endosteal cell by α-irradiation. Killing is balanced by replacement of killed endosteal cells by normal stem cells. This model provides the following interesting predictions for the human ^{224}Ra cases.

1. After the decay of ^{224}Ra the tumor rate decreases exponentially at a rate proportional to the bone turnover rate.

* Work performed under the auspices of the United States Energy Research and Development Administration.

2. For exposure to the same dose the model predicts an increased number of tumors for protracted exposure (i.e. exposure at a lower dose rate).

Implications of this model for the therapy of ankylosing spondylitis are discussed. Statistical procedures are suggested for comparison of this theoretical model with the existing data on the induction of osteosarcomas by ^{224}Ra in man.

INTRODUCTION

Many investigators have attempted to model carcinogenesis in general and radiation in particular. A thorough review of these attempts has been given by Armitage and Doll (1961). Advances in the understanding of the metabolism of radium isotopes (Marshall et al. 1972) and the determination of the cells at risk (Loutit et al. 1967) made it possible to formulate at the cellular level a new mathematical model for osteosarcoma induction in man by α-irradiation (Marshall and Groer 1976). This model was applied successfully of the human ^{226}Ra cases. In this paper we will derive predictions which follow from these equations and will point out possible implications for the treatment of ankylosing spondylitis by ^{224}Ra injections. We will also present a method of statistical analysis of the data on tumor induction by ^{224}Ra in man with specific consideration of competing risks; such an analysis is necessary for a correct comparison of the model with the data.

THE MATHEMATICAL MODEL

The complete set of equations given earlier (Marshall and Groer 1976) is:

$$\begin{aligned}
\dot{M}_0 &= \rho\,(s - \sum_{i=0}^{2} M_i) - F\kappa M_0 - F\sigma M_0 \\
\dot{M}_1 &= F\sigma M_0 - F\kappa M_1 - F\sigma M_1 \\
\dot{M}_2 &= F\sigma M_1 - F\kappa M_2 - \lambda M_2 \qquad (1)\\
\dot{M}_3 &= \lambda M_2
\end{aligned}$$

where M_0 = number of normal endosteal cells ($\sim 10^{11}$);

M_1 = number of endosteal cells initiated once ($\sim 10^5$);

M_2 = number of endosteal cells initiated twice (dormant tumor cells) (0-10);

M_3 = number of promoted tumor cells (0-1);

s = initial number of normal endosteal cells (i.e. $M\ (t = 0) = s$);

κ = killing probability per cell (10^{-2} rad^{-1});

ρ = rate at which killed cells are replaced by M_0 cells (about 0.1 day^{-1});

σ = initiation probability per cell ($\sim 10^{-8}$ rad^{-1});

λ = promotion rate (10^{-2} year^{-1});

F = endosteal dose rate (about 3.2 to about 63 rad day^{-1}).

Figure 1 illustrates the process of tumor induction as described by Eqs. (1). Normal endosteal cells (M_0 cells) can be killed (κ term) or initiated (σ term). If initiated once they become M_1 cells. These cells can be initiated again (M_1 cells become M_2 cells) or some of these cells can be killed. M_2 cells can again be killed, or promoted at a rate λ. We postulate that λ is proportional to the bone turnover rate. The loss of endosteal cells (M_0, M_1, and M_2) through killing is compensated by the first term in the first equation. This term describes the replacement of killed cells by normal stem cells. Killing of M_3 cells has been neglected for two reasons. First, new malignant cells will probably be produced so quickly that only a small proportion could be killed, and second, the tumor cells will soon grow out into the marrow space so that most of the malignant tumor cells will be beyond the range of α-particles emitted from the bone. An estimate for the endosteal dose in the human ^{224}Ra cases can be obtained by multiplying the average skeletal dose by a factor of 9 (Spiess and Mays 1973). This agrees with the endosteal dose derived by Marshall et al. (1974) despite some differences in the derivation of this factor. If one divides this endosteal dose by the injection span one obtains the average endosteal dose rate (Spiess and Mays 1973). For a constant dose rate F, the equations (1) can

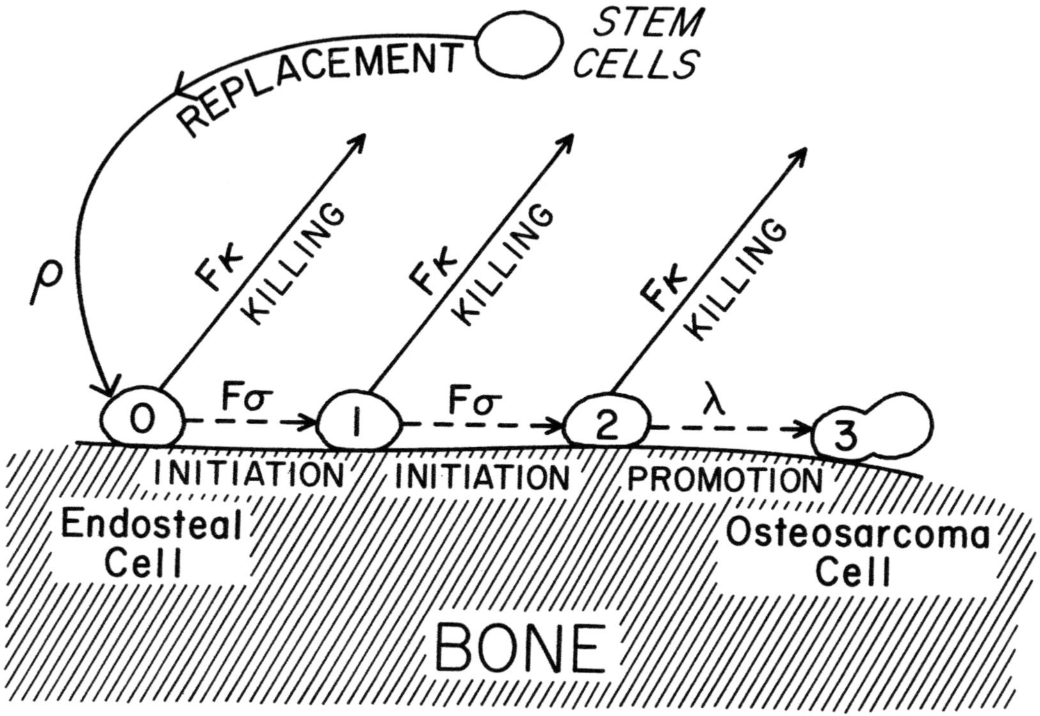

FIGURE 1

Summary of the model. The different events in the tumor induction process as described by Eq. (1) are shown. The numbers indicate the cell type M_0, M_1, M_2 and M_3.

be solved successively and explicitly. We skip the solutions for M and M and give only the solution for the tumor rate P:

$$P\ (t+g) = \lambda M_2\ (t) \quad (2)$$

$$P\ (t+g) \simeq |\rho/(\rho + \kappa F)|\ (\sigma^2\lambda s/\kappa^2)\ |1 - \exp\ (-\kappa Ft) - \kappa Ft\ \exp\ (-\kappa Ft)|$$

where g = tumor growth period (about 5.4 yrs in man (Groer and Marshall 1976)).

Equation (2) is valid for $6 \leq t_d$ (the duration of the injections) and for $\kappa F >> \lambda$ which is certainly the case for the ^{224}Ra cases. The order of magnitude of λ is a few per cent per year and κF for the lowest dose rate in the adult subgroup of the ^{224}Ra cases is about 3% per day. For times larger than the injection period t_d one obtains:

$$P\ (t+g) \simeq |\rho/(\rho + \kappa F)|\ (\sigma^2\lambda s/\kappa^2)\ |1 - \exp\ (-\kappa Ft_d) - \kappa Ft_d\ \exp\ (-\kappa Ft_d)|\ \times \exp\ |-\lambda\ (t - t_d)| \quad (3)$$

PREDICTIONS OF THE MODEL AND METHODS OF COMPARISON WITH THE DATA

Equation (3) shows that after a build-up of M_2 cells during t_d, the number of M_2 cells decreases exponentially. This means that the model predicts a tumor rate $P = \dot{M}_3 \sim \exp\ (-\lambda t)$. It is clear that λ can not be much larger than 0.05 (yr^{-1}) since tumors are still appearing 20 years after the injections. Formula (3) also shows that for the same endosteal dose, lower dose rates will cause more tumors. The ratio R of the number of tumors induced at the lower dose rate, F_L to the number of tumors induced at the higher dose rate F_H is approximately given by:

$$R \simeq (\rho + \kappa F_H)\ /\ (\rho + \kappa F_L) \simeq M_0{}^L\ /\ M_0{}^H \quad (4)$$

where $M_0{}^L$ and $M_0{}^H$ are the number of normal endosteal cells for the two dose rates at the same and otherwise arbitrary time. There are as yet no measurements of the replacement rate ρ available. However, as a first approximation R can be taken to be equal to the observed incidences for the adult long and short span cases (Table 4 in Spiess and Mays 1973). This yields $\rho \simeq 0.175$ (day^{-1}). This implies that on the average every killed cell (M_0, M_1, or M_2) is replaced by a normal cell after approximately 6 days.

If comparative medical follow-up studies should show that the benefits of ^{224}Ra treatment for ankylosing spondylitis outweigh the risks of such a treatment, the following suggestions for ^{224}Ra therapy would follow from the model:

1. The injection spans should be kept as short as feasible. The radiation dose would then be delivered at a higher dose rate and the tumor rate would be lowered as shown by equations (3) and (4).
2. The promotion rate should be kept as small as possible. Since in the model λ is proportional to the bone turnover rate, any treatment in addition to the ^{224}Ra injections which would increase the metabolic activity of bone should be avoided.

These suggestions are a logical consequence of the model considered here and should not be understood as an endorsement of ^{224}Ra therapy. However, these suggestions should be useful for the therapist, if a careful analysis of the data on tumor induction by ^{224}Ra should verify these predictions of the model and if medical follow-up studies should demonstrate the advantage of ^{224}Ra therapy.

The data on tumor induction by ^{224}Ra in adults and children as published in the literature so far does not permit us to make a statistically rigorous comparison of model and data. The reason is the notorious problem of competing risks. The subjects in every medical follow-up study die from many different causes; some are lost from the study and sometimes the study is terminated at an early time when many of the individuals are still alive and well. For this reason the times of death from causes other than osteosarcomas, the times when some individuals were lost from the study and the truncation point of the follow-up are necessary for a rigorous comparison. These times will subsequently be called censoring times as is conventional in statistical analysis. Such an analysis has to be based on the 'model of potential survival times' (see e.g. David 1974) until approaches for interdependent risks have been developed. This model assumes that the different risks (i.e. causes of death) act independently of each other. One cause of death does not influence the potential time of death due to another cause. This assumption of independent risks makes the following analysis of the complete ^{224}Ra data possible.

The tumor rate as given by Eq. (3) defines a time dependent Poisson process. The likelihood of a set of tumor appearance times and censoring times corresponding to a certain cohort of people can therefore be calculated. Simplifying Eq. (3) for the moment we write:

$$P(t) \simeq \lambda B \exp(-\lambda t) \qquad (5)$$

where B is the λ independent factor in equation (3). Time is now measured from the end of the injection period and the tumor growth period g (5.4 years) has been subtracted from all tumor appearance times t_i (i = 1, 2...r) and the censoring times T_i (i = 1, 2...n-r). Equation (5) gives the following cumulative probability distribution:

$$W(t) = 1 - \exp \left| - \int_0^t P(t')\, dt' \right| \qquad (6)$$

where W(t) is the probability of a tumor appearance at a time smaller or equal to t.

The derivative of W(t) is the probability density function w(t). It gives the probability of a tumor appearing in the infinitesimal interval (t, t + dt). The likelihood L of observing a particular set of tumor appearance times t_i and censoring times T_i is given by the following product of probabilities:

$$L = w(t_1)w(t_2)\ldots w(t_r)\left|1 - W(T_1)\right|\left|1 - W(T_2)\right|\ldots\left|1 - W(T_{n-r})\right|$$

Using expressions (5) and (6) the explicit form of the likelihood L can be calculated. One finds for the logarithm of L:

$$\log L = r \log \lambda + r \log B - \lambda \sum_{i=1}^{r} t_i - nB +$$
$$+ B \left(\sum_{i=1}^{r} \exp(-\lambda t_i) + \sum_{i=1}^{n-r} \exp(-\lambda T_i) \right) \qquad (7)$$

Taking the derivative of (7) with respect to λ and setting it equal to zero gives an equation for λ, whose solution is a maximum likelihood estimate for this parameter. ρ can be estimated by comparing the tumor rates soon after the end of the injection period for different dose rates. Knowing these two parameters the expected number of tumors and observed number of tumors can be compared with statistical tests or with a hazard plot (Groer and Marshall 1976).

With the estimated values λ and ρ inserted into Eq. (3), one can then calculate the net risk (see e.g. Chiang 1968) for tumor induction by ^{224}Ra in a given population. This is the risk of an osteosarcoma in a certain time interval after a given injection of ^{224}Ra, if this is the only risk in effect in this population. This net risk can then be used to calculate the number of tumors in an actual population with the appropriate life table. As a corollary of this method of data analysis we would also like to point out, that the net risks should be used when comparing toxicities of different radio nuclides. A simple comparison of cumulative incidences in populations with widely varying survival characteristics is misleading since it does not separate the different risks competing for the life of an individual.

REFERENCES

1. Armitage P. and R. Doll, Stochastic Models for Carcinogenesis. Proc. of the 4th Berkeley Symp. on Math. Statistics and Probability. Vol. 4, p. 19-38 (1961).
2. Chiang, Ch.L., Introduction to Stochastic Processes in Biostatistics, John Wiley & Sons, Inc. New York.

3. David, H.A., Parametric Approaches to the Theory of Competing Risks. Reliability and Biometry, Statistical Analysis of Life Length. F. Proschan and R.J. Serfling (Eds.), SIAM, Philadelphia. p. 275-290 (1974).
4. Groer, P.G. and J.H. Marshall, Hazard Plotting and Estimates for the Tumor Rate and the Tumor Growth Time for Radiogenic Osteosarcomas in Man. Radiological and Environmental Research Division Annual Report, Part II, July 1975-June 1976, ANL 76-88, Part II, Argonne Nat.Lab.Argonne, Illinois 1976.
5. Loutit, J. et al., A Review of the Radiosensitivity of the Tissues in Bone, ICRP Publication 11, Pergamon Press, London 1967.
6. Marshall, J.H. et al., Alkaline Earth Metabolism in Adult Man. ICRP Publication 20, Pergamon Press, New York 1972.
7. Marshall, J.H. et al., Dose to Endosteal Cells and Relative Distribution Factors for ^{224}Ra and ^{239}Pu Compared to ^{226}Ra. Symposium of Biological Effects of ThX, Alta, Utah, July 22-44 (1974).
8. Marschall, J.H. and P.G. Groer, Theory of the Induction of Bone Cancer by Alpha Radiation. Submitted to Radiation Research (1976).
9. Spiess, H. and C.W. Mays, Bone Cancers Induced by ^{224}Ra (ThX) in Children and Adults. Health Physics 19, 713 (1970).
10. Spiess, H. and C.W. Mays, Protraction Effects on Bone Sarcoma Induction of ^{224}Ra in Children and Adults. Radionuclide Carcinogenesis, G.L. Sanders et al. (Eds.) p. 437 (1973).

Methodological aspect of epidemiological inquiries in clinical radiobiology

J. Martin and A. Bertrand

Section d'Informatique et Statistiques Médicales
Groupe INSERM U 115 B.P. 1080 F-54019 NANCY CEDEX
Service de Médecine Nucléaire C. H. U. Brabois
54500 VANDOEUVRE

APPLICATION TO USERS OF ^{224}RA

The difficulty of epidemiological studies in clinical radiobiology is mainly due to:

- determination of the dose effectively delivered to all or part of an organism, especially when there is a radioactive link (localisation and percentage of each isotope, fraction of the dose over a period of time);
- the delay between application of the product and its long-term effects;
- interaction with the spontaneous course and various treatments;
- the relative rareness of complications, the patients are treated from an average age of at least 40 years, after verification of the inefficacy of other treatments.

From a statistical point of view, one should consider that:

- diseases liable to be treated in this way are relatively rare and thus their frequency and that of their complications are estimated with a high degree of variance;
- from one country to another, the positive criteria of the disease and supervision of its course may be different (disparity of international terminology). It is thus difficult to obtain a homogeneous sample;

- it is not possible, except retrospectively, to study control groups.

Consequently, in any epidiomical study of this field, it is necessary to obtain the agreement of specialists of numerous countries on objective criteria of definition of the disease and its stages to permit comparison of comparable things.

- not to loose sight of any patients for we are seeking events of low probability on groups with necessarily restricted numbers.

RECOMMENDATIONS

Consequently, it appears that recommendations may be proposed by the working group on the use of ^{224}Ra if the latter should continue to be used in man.

1. Any specialist requesting ^{224}Ra, should undertake to transmit and fill in a pre-drawn up clinical record sheet, according to criteria of recognition defining precisely the disease and its course. It would be a good thing if suppliers of ^{224}Ra only delivered this substance to laboratories who accept these conditions and respect them.
2. The treated patient must be warned that this treatment requires strict supervision and undertake to accept regular consultations for supervision and reply to questionnaires periodically.
3. All these data are centralised as soon as they are received by an independent research group which undertakes the work of analysis and synthesis. Regular information is given in return on the results of this permanent inquiry. This group also keeps up to date the card index system in liaison with the supplier.

We are prepared to undertake this work if it is possible to obtain agreement on all the previous points and the latter.

Notre expérience du ^{224}Ra dans le traitement de la spondylarthrite ankylosante

H. Roux, A. Schiano, D. Kiprandi, G. Serratrice
et R. Paulin, F. Roux

Clinique Rhumatologique,
C.H.U. Timone, Av. Jean Moulin - Marseille, France
Service Central de Médecine Nucléaire
C.H.U. Timone, Av. Jean Moulin - Marseille, France

SUMMARY

The efficiency of ^{224}Ra in the treatment of ankylosing spondylitis is confirmed in 39 patients who were not responsive to usual treatment or could not be treated thus.
With lower doses relapses are more frequent but side effects (clinical and biological) are less numerous.

L'effet thérapeutique du ^{224}Ra dans la spondylarthrite ankylosante est connu depuis d'un demi-siècle, mais la possibilité d'accidents avec les premières préparations a limité son usage en France. Depuis 1960, le ^{224}Ra n'a été utilisé qu'à Nancy et Marseille et actuellement, à Marseille seulement.

MATERIEL ET METHODES

Nous avons traité 39 patients (36 hommes, 3 femmes) âgés de 32 à 75 ans présentant des localisations axiales, 10 d'entre eux seulement présentaient également des manifestations périphériques. Ces malades étaient tous porteurs de spondylarthrite ankylosante grave, résistante aux anti-inflammatoires usuels, ou présentant des contre-indications à ces médicaments (ulcère gastro duodénal), hémorragies digestives etc.). Deux protocoles thérapeutiques ont été utilisés: chez 17 patients, les injections intraveineuses de ^{224}Ra ont été pratiquées tous les quinze jours, avec des posologies croissantes, jusqu'à une dose totale moyenne de 1000 µCi; chez les 22 autres malades, la dose totale moyenne obtenue par des posologies constantes tous les quinze jours, n'a été que de 500 µCi.

RESULTATS

L'effet thérapeutique est considéré avec un recul de 6 à 36 mois. Dans les deux groupes, l'efficacité thérapeutique concerne essentiellement les déterminations axiales et se situe au même niveau. Cependant les rechutes sont plus fréquentes et apparaissent plus précocément avec les doses totales les plus faibles.

La vitesse de sédimentation diminue moins souvent avec les faibles doses mais les effets secondaires sont plus nombreux et plus importants avec les fortes doses. En particulier, une diminution du nombre des érythrocytes, des leucocytes et des plaquettes sanguines, apparaît de façon plus importante avec ces fortes doses.

CONCLUSIONS

Ce travail confirme l'efficacité du ^{224}Ra et les résultats obtenus dans 39 spondylarthrites ankylosantes pour lesquelles les traitements habituels sont inefficaces ou contre-indiqués, se révèlent particulièrement intéressants. Avec les faibles doses, les rechutes sont plus fréquentes, mais les effets secondaires, cliniques et biologiques, sont plus rares qu'avec les fortes doses.

TABLE

	Résultats ininter-prétables	Resultats cliniques				Rechutes
		Très bons	Bons	Moyens	Echecs	
1er Groupe: Doses progressives jusqu'à un total de 448 à 1300 μCi 17 patients	1	10	2	1	3	1
2e Groupe: Doses constantes jusqu'à un total de 280 à 560 μCi 22 patients	2	9	6	2	3	4 (après 6 mois)

Round table discussion I
Risk evaluation of ankylosing spondylitis therapy

Moderator, C.W. Mays

References giving additional information
have been inserted (in brackets).

J. Martin: Is it possible that some of the effects seen with ^{224}Ra treatment are due to long-lived α-emitter contamination?

O. Delikan: There are no significant amounts of long-lived contaminants in the ^{224}Ra, prepared by the Buchler Firm since 1949. (See the paper by Delikan in this symposium for more details. Also, the analysis by Spiess and Mays, Health Physics 19, pp. 713-729 (1970), indicates that for the patients injected since 1944, the skeletal dose from the contaminants was negligible compared to that from ^{224}Ra.)

K.R. Trott: What is the expected number of bone sarcoma cases in the treated ankylosing spondylitis patients?

C.W. Mays: Thank you, Dr. Trott, for giving me the opportunity to discuss the predictions I presented here 3 years ago at Professor Hug's 60th birthday (Health Physics 25, pp. 585-592 (1973)). At that time, the follow-up by Dr. Schales had started, and I estimated that he could trace 1000-2000 ankylosing spondylitis patients in the low dose range below 90 rad. These adult patients typically received a total of 280 µCi ^{224}Ra in 10 fractions with a week between each injection, and their calculated average skeletal doses were 56 rads. The following risk estimates were based on various dose response models fit to the Spiess adults.

PREDICTED 20-YEAR RISK FROM CURRENT TREATMENT

(56 rads av.skel. dose to spondylitic adults)

Dose-response model	Predicted bone sarcomas / 1000 patients
Linear	5
(Linear) x (injection span factor)	3
(Dose squared) x (exponential)	2
Threshold below 90 rad	0

If one takes the simple linear model and ignores the protraction effect, 5 bone sarcomas would be expected among 1000 patients. But, if one modifies the linear coefficient by an injection span factor, 3 bone sarcomas are predicted. On the other hand, if one assumes, as Drs. Groer and Marshall have (see their paper in this symposium), that two radiation events are required to initiate the cancer, then there would be a dose-squared initiation. Multiplying the dose-squared initiation by an exponential to allow for cell killing, 2 cases are predicted. Finally, if a threshold exists below an average skeletal dose of 90 rad, then zero cases should be induced by doses below the threshold. The predicted risk to an individual receiving the current therapy is between 0 and 0.5%.

W.A. Müller: The real results up to now, are 418 deaths, but no osteosarcomas below 90 rad. This would support the threshold model.

C.W. Mays: I must point out that while Dr. Schales was able to trace somewhat over 1000 patients below 90 rads, many of these patients were recently injected and have not yet survived 20 years. Future bone sarcomas may still occur in these patients.

W. Koch: We have treated about 900 ankylosing spondylitis patients since 1948, with follow-up in 1951, 1953, 1957, 1964, and now, again, from 1973 to 1976, as suggested by, and in collaboration with Dr. Schales. During this time, we have not seen a single case of osteosarcomas in these patients and, also, we have recorded no death as a result of osteosarcoma. I would like to make the supplementary comment that it would already approach a little closer those percentages of 0-0.5% which you have mentioned, however, with the reservation that, naturally, all cases should be at least looked at over a time span of up to 25 years.

W. Gössner: What now are the number of oldest cases?

W. Koch: I have about 200 cases which have been followed for 25 years.

C.W. Mays: I have a question. Maybe you can help. Some months ago, I received a letter from Dr. Schales stating that one of the patients in his follow-up had a reticulum cell sarcoma of the bone marrow. I had intended to ask him more details on this patient, but that is not possible now.

W.A. Müller: I hope we can find this patient. (This patient's average skeletal dose was probably between 60 and 112 rads. For details see the paper, Risk to bone from present ^{224}therapy, by C.W. Mays in this symposium.)

H. Spiess: I don't believe in a threshold because bone sarcomas have occurred at 10 to 20 rads in the Thorotrast patients.

W.A. Müller: Although there are many osteosarcomas in the radium dial painters, it seems like a threshold exists because there are no osteosarcomas in the many persons below about 900 rads from ^{226}Ra.

P.G. Groer: A threshold really can never be established by experiment because wherever the threshold seems to be, there is always a lower possibility. The model I presented today is not a threshold one. The reason, I believe, why we see this 'funny' threshold effect at Argonne, is that we have a limited population. If we had an infinite population, we would see tumors at lower doses.

R.H. Mole: I agree with everything that Dr. Groer said, except his last phrase. You can't know that if you had a larger population you would have found tumors at lower doses. You can expect it, but you can't know it.

C.W. Mays: There are at least 28 dial painters who died

with bone sarcomas, but whose doses have not yet been evaluated (A.T. Keane et al., Radiat.Res. 67, pp. 625-626 (1976)). It is premature to conclude that none of their sarcomas occurred below 900 rads from long-lived radium.

R.H. Mole: I may lose all the friends I have, but I have an important criticism of all the 3 speakers this morning, you (Mays) included.

C.W. Mays: Well, if you put it that way, I can't say no.

R.H. Mole: You put a great deal on the existence of a protraction factor in the Spiess human data, but I would remind you, it doesn't exist. Dose goes up with protraction and so does the incidence per rad. That means you have a square dose response. There might be a protraction factor, but I don't think your evidence allows one to conclude this from the data in man.

C.W. Mays: We were quite aware that the dose tends to increase with the number of injections. Therefore, we divided each dose group into two subgroups of longer and shorter injection span, but roughly equal dose. Then we combined the longer span subgroups and, also, the shorter span subgroups with the following result (see H. Spiess and C.W. Mays, in Radionuclide Carcinogenesis, USAEC CONF-720505, pp. 437-450 (1973)). Holding the dose relatively constant, the observed incidence was greater with the longer injection span, both in juveniles and in adults, in good agreement with that calculated from our protraction effect equations.

R.H. Mole: Yes, but there is no statistically established difference.

SIMILAR DOSES BUT VARIABLE SPANS

	Doses (rads)	Spans (months)	Calculated % incidence	Observed % incid. ± S.D.
Juveniles	1100	15.6	19.4	20.2 ± 3.9
	1110	6.8	13.5	13.5 ± 3.3
Adults	217	10.4	2.5	2.3 ± 0.9
	209	4.3	1.6	1.6 ± 0.7

C.W. Mays: You are perfectly right that in these human data taken alone, the difference is suggestive ($P = 0.16$) rather than statistically significant, so maybe we are friends again. The conclusive evidence that a protraction effect exists, comes from the well-controlled experiments in mice, here at Neuherberg, where the total ^{224}Ra dose was held constant, while the protraction span was varied. For a constant total dose, the incidence of bone sarcomas increased with protraction span. The statistics on the Neuherberg results are much better and give experimental validity to what the available human data could only suggest.

R.H. Mole: But protraction is not a scientific concept. You must have some idea of mechanism before you can transfer from animal to man.

W.A. Müller: Comparability of animal and human data is one of the items for our discussion. What about thresholds or safe doses for different animal species and humans? Maybe we should discuss this in connection with protraction.

C.W. Mays: I recently plotted the best data I could find on bone sarcoma induction by α-emitters, and list them here under three groupings: Those in which the dose-response at low dose appeared to be approximately linear; those concave upward; and those concave downward (C.W. Mays et al., in: Health Effects of Plutonium, J.W. Press, University of Utah, pp. 343-362 (1976)).

Let me say a few words about each. The first example is the Spiess patients in the dose range 0-1000 rads with a protraction factor. The ^{239}Pu results are from our own beagles. The week before I left, one of our lowest-dose ^{239}Pu beagles died with a bone sarcoma at an average skeletal dose of only 2.3 rads, and another, from the same group, recently died with an epidermoid carcinoma of the frontal sinus at an average of only 2.4 rads. Numbers like these make me believe that if there is a threshold for plutonium, it is so low that for practical purposes, it does not exist. ^{228}Th is a bone surface seeker, like

BONE SARCOMA INDUCTION vs. α-DOSE

(indications as of 1975)

APPROXIMATELY LINEAR

1. ^{224}Ra in humans 0-1000 rad (Spiess and Mays 1973)
2. ^{239}Pu in beagles 0-140 rad (Mays et al. 1976)
3. ^{228}Th in beagles 0-320 rad (Mays, unpublished)
4. ^{239}Pu in rats 0-100 rad (Buldakov et al. 1970)
5. ^{226}Ra in mice 0-500 rad (M. Finkel et al. 1969)
6. ^{227}Th in mice 0-200 rad (Luz et al. 1976)
7. ^{239}Pu in mice 0-1000 rad (Mays et al.11976)

CONCAVE UPWARDS

1. ^{226}Ra and ^{228}Ra in man 0-2000 rad (Rowland and Stehney 1974)
2. ^{226}Ra in beagles 0-2500 rad (Mays et al. 1976)
3. ^{228}Ra in beagles 0-800 rad (Mays, unpublished)

CONCAVE DOWNWARDS

1. ^{224}Ra in mice 0-150 rad (Luz et al. 1976)

^{239}Pu, and in beagles, its response, also, appears to be linear at low doses. ^{239}Pu in rats, ^{226}Ra in Miriam Finkel's mice, ^{227}Th in the Neuherberg mice, and ^{239}Pu in our mice seem to give approximately linear responses at low doses.

The existing data for the United States radium dial painters support a concave upward dose response. So did the ^{226}Ra and ^{228}Ra data in our beagles, at the time I prepared this slide. But about a month ago, a new osteosarcoma occurred at a lower dose-level of ^{226}Ra than ever previously, so that, now, the ^{224}Ra dose-response curve in beagles can be regarded either as approximately linear or only slightly concave upwards.

The one well documented example of a concave downward response is for single injections of ^{224}Ra in the Neuherberg mice.

R.H. Mole: In the people with ^{226}Ra, how much dose is wasted because the tumour has already started?

C.W. Mays: The dose received in about the last 5 years before death.

R.H. Mole: How do you know?

C.W. Mays: Because volume doubling times of 19 to 72 days have been measured in 6 human bone sarcomas (J.S. Spratt, The rates of growth of skeletal sarcomas, Cancer 18, pp. 14-25 (1965)). It requires 40 volume doubling times for a tumor to enlarge from a diameter of 0.001 cm (the size of a typical tumor cell) to a diameter of 10 cm (the size of a typical human tumor at death). So assuming the volume doubling time for a bone sarcoma in an individual remains fairly constant, the individual growth periods in man ranged from about 2 to 8 years. We have measured the growth rates of 249 osteosarcomas in beagles, and in only one case did the assumption of a constancy of doubling time throughout tumor growth lead to the unrealistic conclusion that the tumor was induced before the radioactivity was injected (G.B. Thurman et al., Growth 35, pp. 119-124 (1971)).

P.G. Groer: What is meant by 'latent period'?

R.H. Mole: Some people use it for the interval between treatment and the mean appearance time of the tumors. That's a very confusing definition. Others use it in the mystical sense to imply the period during which something unknown is going on in the body before the tumor begins to grow. But since you never know when the tumor starts growing, I think we shouldn't use this last definition.

P.G. Groer: Many investigators take it as the time from the start of irradiation to the appearance of the first tumor. But if you don't state the population at risk, this is meaningless. If the population were 10 times larger, the first tumor would probably come earlier.

C.W. Mays: This is likely. In the Spiess series, the shortest appearance time for bone sarcomas was 3.5 years among some 200 children. If there had been 2000 children, perhaps it would been 3 years: If there had been 2 million children, perhaps only 2 years.

P.G. Groer: That's so.

C.W. Mays: Our time is almost gone. Dr. Spiess, you have been rather quiet, so I would like you to summarize what you think is the most important thing that has been said during this discussion.

H. Spiess: I think the most important thing for me is that we don't know if there is any threshold for ^{224}Ra.

Round table discussion II
Clinical results of ankylosing spondylitis therapy

Moderator, W. Koch

Koch: First of all I would like to make some fundamental remarks regarding the three different manifestations of ankylosing spondylitis in their various stages. My exposition is based on the clinical and roentgenographic evaluation of more than 2000 patients treated at our hospital. One has to distinguish between the painful inflammatory type of ankylosing spondylitis and the purely osseous one. The majority of cases, i.e. about two thirds, represent a mixed form where inflammatory and osseous processes affect different segments of the spine alternatively or even at the same time. Depending on the symptom of pain, the disease is diagnosed *early* as 'Bechterew' in the purely inflammatory cases and also in the mixed form, while the purely osseous type will be diagnosed *late*, usually when the spine is already stiff. In each of these three types we find the following different phases of the disease, classified according to the clinical and roentgenographic manifestations:

Phase I: Involvement of the iliosacral joint only as iliosacral arthritis

Phase II: Involvement of the iliosacral joint and of the lumbar spine

Phase III: Involvement of the iliosacral joint, of the lumbar and thoracic spine

Phase IV: Involvement of the iliosacral joint, of the lumbar, thoracic, and cervical spine.

These four phases will not necessarily be reached in

all cases of ankylosing spondylitis, but the disease can be arrested in phase I, II, or III. In about 30 per cent of all ankylosing spondylitis patients of the three different types mentioned, passing or lasting involvement of the joints at the extremities has been observed. Due to the long follow-up time of our patients I was able to point out already in 1968 that in dependent on the different course of the disease the osseous stiffening of the spine is not always arrested after ^{224}Ra therapy when the osseous involvement is the predominant one. An arrest in the phase II or III can probably be better explained by the mainly inflammatory involvement in a case belonging to the mixed type. The decisive criterion for the Bechterew patient is the observation that ^{224}Ra treatment is followed by a long period without or at least allivated pain where he does not need antirheumatic drugs.

I would like to ask Mr. Windeyer whether he administers X-ray therapy also in dependence on the course of the disease as described before or just in dependence on the diagnosis 'Bechterew'?

Windeyer: I think I am in difficulties here because I haven't recognized these three manifestations of the disease. We have believed that it is one disease and that it stops in the majority of cases at an early age. The youngest patient I have ever seen was 15, but I think the majority is around the twenties. The problem for me is whether the older age groups with calcification of the intervertebral ligaments and a greater proportion of proliferous involvement have in fact started a good deal earlier and have not been recognized so that I have not appreciated these three manifestations of the disease. We have not differentiated between a type which is predominantly inflammatory and one of predominantly osseous involvement, but have treated the patients when the diagnosis of ankylosing spondilitis had been made and when the disease was reactive.

Koch: In reply to Mr. Windeyer I like to remark that in

the first years after 1948 we have also treated all patients with ^{224}Ra whenever the diagnosis was verified. Only after a long-term follow-up of our patients we came to differentiate between the three manifestations of ankylosing spondylitis in their various phases, and this helped us to decide upon the indication for ^{224}Ra treatment in each individual case. It reduced the number of patients who got ^{224}Ra treatment, and by this, I believe, we also reduced possible radiation hazards which must be thought about also when treating grown-ups with ^{224}Ra, according to the exposition of Mr. Spiess et al.

Now I like to ask Mr. Hartl to report on his results.

Schmitt: He has treated about 30 patients with ^{224}Ra. Among those were 20-24 who said that they felt immediately better after the treatment with ^{224}Ra.

Koch: Our French colleagues Martin and Bertrand said that the ^{224}Ra dosage which they apply is twice as high as the one we use since 1950 and which amounts to a total of 280 μCi. Only between 1948 and 1959 we used a dosage as high as the French one. Our follow-up studies of up to 25 years after the first ^{224}Ra treatment showed that progression of the spine stiffening does not depend on the ^{224}Ra dosage but rather on the mainly osseous and less inflammatory involvement in a particular case of ankylosing spondylitis. Thus we have seen patients who were treated in another hospital with 2800 μCi, which is 10 times as much as we use, and yet the total spine had become stiff. We find that a higher dosage than 280 μCi is not justified because an arrest of the ossification process cannot be induced in each case. An arrest or delay of the ossification process depends rather on the manifestation of the disease and its actual phase.

Müller: I would like to ask Mr. Roux about the follow-up period of his patients.

Roux: The longest is 3 years; altogether between 6 months and 3 years.

Trott: What is the best to do for a doctor who has a patient with a Bechterew? There are three ways: give them drugs.

But the old drugs are very toxic and may have late toxic effects. The new drugs are so new that we don't know anything about their late toxic effects yet. It is very likely that they have some on the kidney and so on. So we cannot judge the risks associated with these drugs. Then there is the question: external or internal radiotherapy? From the data of the old external radiotherapy I gathered that among 14000 patients there are 60 cases of leukemia. And because of these 60 cases the treatment has nearly been stopped, or at least has been very much reduced. If I got the figures of Mr. Windeyer right, the present-day radiotherapy is about half the dosage to less than half the volume, so one would expect risks from external radiotherapy which were in the order of about 1 of 1000 patients treated with a very effective therapy which causes immediate relief of pain and necessitates no further drugs. We don't know whether the ^{224}Ra carries a risk which is higher or lower, at least it is probably not very much higher than this. If it is lower we don't know, but I think some people in the audience believe it is about the same or could be about the same. So from what I learned at this meeting I would say, if I had a patient I would recommend him straightforward X-ray therapy after the old data. I don't see any evidence presented in the whole meeting which indicates that this is worse than the other more risky treatment and I think that it is still the most efficient way. What do you think, Mr. Koch and Mr. Windeyer, about this, how would you answer a young doctor who is going to start a therapy?

Windeyer: I would like refer to what Mr. Martin has said about follow-up. Can we afford to follow-up every type of patient who is treated in the hospital? In my country it is impossible because it costs a high amount of money to do this. We did it in some cases. As far as it concerns the ankylosing spondylitis we do the follow-up on all patients after radiotherapy because of the leukemia point of view. This is how Sir Brian Doll got his 14532 cases and my 1400 are part of those. We do know that that follow-up was very complete and that the figures I showed you now 13 years after the treatment contained no cases of bone sarcoma among the 14000.

Mays: But there were 5 cases of bone sarcoma which had been treated with ^{224}Ra in the years between 1957 and 1967.

Spiess: Before Mr. Koch answers to this question, my question to Mr. Windeyer: Do you recommend the X-ray treatment?

Windeyer: I don't know anything about the treatment with ^{224}Ra. So I am keeping to that subject I know something about, and I said already yesterday at the end of my paper, if I would suffer myself, I would give serious consideration to the method of treatment which I know would be effective. This may increase my normal expectation developing leukemia by 10 times, but this is in fact only one third of one per cent, and I think that is a fair risk to take.

Mole: There is quite satisfying evidence in the older literature, derived from controlled trials, that X-ray treatment of ankylosing spondylitis can be beneficial without, however, completely arresting the ankylosing process. The best long-term results are, therefore, achieved by combining X-ray treatment with systematic measures of other kinds (Sharp, J. and E.C. Easson. British Medical J. I, 619-623 (1954)).

Local X-ray treatment of joints in patients with 'rheumatoid arthritis' could produce subjective benefit, but objective improvement which could be attributed to the treatment was slight. The chief and not very common symptomatic improvement was decrease in pain and this was often psychogenic in origin (Smyth, C.J., R.H. Freyberg and W.S. Peck. J.American Medical Assoc. 116, 1995-2001 (1941)). In contrast the same investigators found that about three quarters of the cases of spondylitis rhizomélique, 'rheumatoid arthritis of the spine', given X-ray treatment of the spine were significantly improved as judged by physical examination. The improvement rate was higher in patients with early disease (Smyth et al., Smyth, C.J., R.H. Freyberg and I. Lampe. J.American Medical

Assoc. 117, 826-830 (1941)).

Koch: Before starting a treatment with ^{224}Ra the diagnosis of ankylosing spondylitis must be verified. This is much easier today since in 95 per cent of all cases the immune biological factor HL-A 27 is positive. During phase I, in iliosacral arthritis, as well as during phases II and III of the purely inflammatory type with involvement of the small vertebral joints it is sufficient to give antirheumatic drugs (Voltaren^R, Indometacin^R, etc.) during the painful stages and to examine the patients every 6-12 months. Only when therapeutic resistance sets in and syndesmophyte formation at the lumbar and thoracic spine is seen in the roentgenogram as well as osseous ankylosis of some of the vertebral joints during phase II and III the ^{224}Ra therapy is indicated. Once the disease has reached phase IV and ossification of the spine is perfect the treatment comes too late. In none of our 695 patients treated with 280 μCi ^{224}Ra it came to a bone sarcoma. Regarding the X-ray therapy in the treatment of ankylosing spondylitis, I have no experiences. I have had patients, though, who had been treated with X-ray but were not free of pain until they got ^{224}Ra.

Trott: For how long will you have to hospitalize a patient for the external radiotherapy and for the internal one? If I get it right, no hospitalization for X-ray therapy, but for internal therapy - how long; I think this is a very big factor for my decision.

Koch: For the internal radiotherapy the patient stays in hospital for 3 months. At the same time physiotherapy is administered. It is important to activate the patient in order to inhibit the ossification process, and that is more successfully done in hospital.

Schmitt: In my collective of patients I have had some who were treatment with X-ray before and then got pains again later. I think everybody uses the therapy with which he has the best experiences. We had that with ^{224}Ra.

Finally it was discussed and agreed on by all participants that the Schales-study - that is a centralized registration and follow-up of all ankylosing spondylitis patients treated with ^{224}Ra - should be continued, and it was recommended that the patient collective of Mr. Martin would be included.

Concluding remarks

R.H. Mole

MRC Radiobiology Unit
Harwell, Didcot, Oxfordshire OX11 ORD, England

It is always difficult, I think, to say something useful after a group of intelligent people have been discussing important questions over a period as long as two days. The important conclusion seems to be: the follow-up studies in the Federal Republic of Germany of patients who have received ^{224}Ra should be continued. Here is a unique opportunity and responsibility which I hope those in the Federal Republic will accept on behalf of those who live in that country and on behalf of everyone wherever they may live. Professor Martin has stressed the difficulties of extracting reliable information about uncommonly occurring events from populations numbering only, say, a thousand. However, information on whether 0, 1, 2 or 3 (or more) bone sarcomas occur in 1000 cases of ankylosing spondylitis treated with ^{224}Ra would be in my opinion very valuable information, both clinically and in the field of public health.

My second impression, after being brought up-to-date on what is now known about ankylosing spondylitis as a clinical entity, is that the time seems ripe for an intensive investigation into this disease in a clinical setting, for instance in a University Department. New and important information, for instance about the association of specific HLA antigens and the disease, is now available. A great deal is known about the treatment of acute diseases and increasingly the medical challenge lies in the chronic and disabling illness, especially those which attack young adults in the prime of life. Ankylosing spondylitis is a complex and strikingly interesting example. I came to this meeting wondering whether radiation treatment truly relieved the pain of this disease and I have been quite convinced by what we have been told. Pain is indeed a subjective phenomenon but good clinical observations are in my view as good scientific evidence as good observations by naturalists in any field. But it is also clear that no mechanism for the relief of pain by radiation is at all well established. Indeed, although no one asked how pain is relieved by anti-inflammatory drugs, that is perhaps just as difficult a question. Although pain is subjective, its severity and relief can be examined scientifically and without bias - for instance, by having an observer who does not know what particular treatment an individual patient has received, a methodology now well established.

I hope that means can be found for support of clinical research into ankylosing spondylitis especially in clinics where ^{224}Ra is used in its treatment. Modern methods applied to patients under treatment would greatly increase our knowledge of the metabolism of ^{224}Ra. It is now a long time since Fritz Schales, whose death we all regret so much, provided the little that we know. This meeting was supported by funds from Euratom and organisations concerned with radiological protection are anxious to learn all they can about the metabolism and effects of ^{224}Ra in man. Surely it would be advantageous to provide support for research in a clinical environment and so help the study both of individual patients and of the long-term outcome of their illness and its treatment.

As Professor Spiess reminded us, ^{224}Ra given to children has caused a distressingly high frequency of bone sarcoma. However, if an excessive quantity of any medicinal agent is used and ill effects occur, that is not necessarily an argument against using that agent in smaller amounts. The surveys of Spies and Mays have provided facts which help considerably in judging what would be a suitably safe total amount of ^{224}Ra to give a patient. It would also be quite wrong, I believe, to think that standards of radiological protection of the general public have any bearing on the choice of treatment for a painful and severely disabling disease. The differentiated follicular thyroid carcinomas are usually much less disabling than ankylosing spondylitis but no one would deny such cases treatment with millicurie amounts of radioactive iodine simply on public health grounds nor because of regulations about radio-pharmaceuticals used for diagnostic purposes. It is an error to lay stress on the possibility of hereditary damage in the children and further descendants of those treated with ^{224}Ra if, as is the case, radium is not concentrated in the gonads and the genetically significant radiation dose is very small.

It is a commonplace of modern medicine that effective therapeutic agents often have important side effects so that in an individual patient the advantages and disadvantages of a given therapy have to be balanced one against the other. If ^{224}Ra in therapeutically effective amounts cause bone sarcoma in just a few of a thousand patients that might well be an acceptable frequency of unwanted damage in the treatment of a serious disease.

We have all missed Professor Otto Hug and, when I spoke to him on the telephone just now, he seemed in warm agreement with the suggestion that clinical research in ankylosing spondylitis would be well worth doing from the point of view of the sick patient as well as from the point of view of public health. I hope you all agree.

In Professor Hug's absence, Professor Gössner has led us admirably and I'm sure you would all wish to join in thanking him and all the other members of this laboratory concerned with this Symposium for the efficiency and friendly atmosphere of the arrangements.

List of participants

Bahous, I.	Rheumatologische Universitätsklinik Burgfeldstr. 101 Basel, Schweiz
Bertrand, A.	Service de Médecine Nucléaire C.H.U. Nancy-Brabois 54500 Vandoeuvre-le-Nancy, France
Delikan, O.	Amersham Buchler GmbH & Co KG Harxbütteler Strasse 3 3300 Braunschweig-Wenden, Deutschland
Dunker, M.	Rheumaklinik Landesbad Aachen Am Burtscheider Markt 24 5100 Aachen, Deutschland
Dolphin, G.W.	National Radiological Protection Board Harwell Didcot Oxfordshire OX11 ORQ, United Kingdom
Ebert, H.G.	Kommission der Europäischen Gemeinschaften Rue de la Loi 200 1040 Brüssel, Belgien
Erfle, V.	Institut für Biologie, Gesellschaft für Strahlen- und Umweltforschung mbH München Ingolstädter Landstrasse 1 8042 Neuherberg, Deutschland
Gössner, W.	Abteilung für Allg.u.Exp. Pathologie, Gesellschaft für Strahlen- und Umweltfor- schung mbH München Ingolstädter Landstrasse 1 8042 Neuherberg, Deutschland
Groer, P.G.	Radiological and Environmental Research Division, Argonne National Laboratory 9700 South Cass Avenue Argonne, Illinois 60439, USA

Hartl, W.	Rheumaklinik Landesbad und Rheumaforschungs-institut Aachen Am Burtscheider Markt 24 5100 Aachen, Deutschland
Jacobi, W.	Institut für Strahlenschutz, Gesellschaft für Strahlen- und Umweltforschung mbH München Ingolstädter Landstrasse 1 8042 Neuherberg, Deutschland
Koch, W.	Orthopädische Klinik und Poliklinik (Hüffer-stiftung) der Westfälischen Wilhelmsuniver-sität Hüfferstrasse 27 4400 Münster/Westfalen, Deutschland
Kofránek, V.	Institute of Hygiene and Epidemiology Department of Radiation Hygiene Srobarova 48 Prague 10, CSSR
Linzner, U.	Abteilung für Strahlenbiol. und Biophysik Gesellschaft für Strahlen- und Umwelt-forschung mbH Ingolstädter Landstrasse 1 8042 Neuherberg, Deutschland
Luz, A.	Abteilung für Allg.u.Exp. Pathologie Gesellschaft für Strahlen- und Umwelt-forschung mbH Ingolstädter Landstrasse 1 8042 Neuherberg, Deutschland
Martin, J.	Service de Médecine Nucléaire C.H.U. Nancy-Brabois 54500 Vandoeuvre-les-Nancy, France
Marquart, K.-H.	Abteilung für Allg.u.Exp. Pathologie Gesellschaft für Strahlen- und Umwelt-forschung mbH Ingolstädter Landstrasse 1 8042 Neuherberg, Deutschland
Mays, C.W.	Dept.of Anatomy and Radiobiological Division College of Medicine, University of Utah Salt Lake City/Utah, USA

Mole, R.H.	Medical Research Center, Radiobiology Unit Harwell Didcot Oxon 0X11 ORD, United Kingdom
Müller, W.A.	Abteilung für Strahlenbiologie u. Biophysik Gesellschaft für Strahlen- und Umwelt- forschung mbH München Ingolstädter Landstrasse 1 8042 Neuherberg, Deutschland
Parchwitz, E.	Institut für Biologie, Gesellschaft für Strahlen- und Umweltforschung mbH München Ingolstädter Landstrasse 1 8042 Neuherberg, Deutschland
Roux, H.	Clinique Rhumatologique, C.H.U. Timone Rue Saint-Pierre 13005 Marseille, France
Schilling, F.	Zentrum für Rheuma-Pathologie Rheinstrasse 4 6500 Mainz, Deutschland
Schmid, A.	Amersham Buchler GmbH & Co KG Harxbütteler Strasse 3 3300 Braunschweig-Wenden, Deutschland
Schmitt, E.	Orthopädische Universitätsklinik und Poli- klinik Friedrichsheim Frankfurt/M. Marienburgstrasse 2 6000 Frankfurt am Main-Niederrad 71, Deutschland
Sonnabend, E.	Universitätsklinik für Zahn-, Mund- und Kieferkrankheiten Goethestrasse 70 8000 München 2, Deutschland
Spiess, H.	Kinderpoliklinik der Universität München Pettenkoferstrasse 8a 8000 München 2, Deutschland
Trott, K.-R.	Strahlenbiologisches Institut der Universi- tät München Bavariaring 19 8000 München 2, Deutschland

Volf, V. Institut für Strahlenbiologie
Kernforschungszentrum Karlsruhe
Postfach 3640
7500 Karlsruhe, Deutschland

Wallner, B. Abteilung für Allg.u.Exp. Pathologie
Gesellschaft für Strahlen- und Umwelt-
forschung mbH München
Ingolstädter Landstrasse 1
8042 Neuherberg, Deutschland

Windeyer, Sir B. Moreton Gap, Thame Park Road
Thame OX9 3PP, United Kingdom

Winkler, C. Institut für klinische und experimentelle
Nuklearmedizin der Universität Bonn
Venusberg
5300 Bonn, Deutschland

Wittenzellner, R. Gesellschaft für Strahlen- und Umwelt-
forschung mbH München
Ingolstädter Landstrasse 1
8042 Neuherberg, Deutschland

GPSR Compliance

The European Union's (EU) General Product Safety Regulation (GPSR) is a set of rules that requires consumer products to be safe and our obligations to ensure this.

If you have any concerns about our products, you can contact us on ProductSafety@springernature.com

In case Publisher is established outside the EU, the EU authorized representative is:

Springer Nature Customer Service Center GmbH
Europaplatz 3
69115 Heidelberg, Germany

Batch number: 10583998

Printed by Printforce, the Netherlands